THE NEW A
AND COMMON SENSE

The New Arthritis and Common Sense

by
Dale Alexander

ILLUSTRATED   •   WITH MENUS

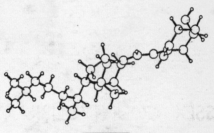

An imprint of William Heinemann Limited

Published by Cedar Books

an imprint of

William Heinemann Limited
10 Upper Grosvenor Street, London W1X 9PA

LONDON   MELBOURNE
JOHANNESBURG   AUCKLAND

First published by The Witkower Press Inc.
West Hartford, Connecticut, USA
Previous edition first published 1957
by World's Work Limited

First published as a Cedar Book 1987

0 434 01819 8

Printed in Great Britain by
Richard Clay Ltd
Bungay, Suffolk

A personal message . . .

from a grateful author . . .

This book could not have been written without the help of one very special person. She is a lady. Her loyal support and her constant encouragement continued through the long months while this manuscript was being written. No words can adequately express my deep appreciation to Ida Rae Fischer.

Illustrations by Florence Valentine-Omens

VITAMIN

D₃

SEE PAGE 36

Throughout this book, the author presents his personal views and observations. His statements and opinions are meant to serve only as an informational guide, hopefully to help prevent disease. Persons who are in ill health should seek medical advice from a doctor, before embarking on any dietary program. Any reader who is taking medicine upon a doctor's prescription should not change nor terminate that medication without consulting a physician. The facts and the diet described in these pages are subject to different interpretations and results. In other words, after reading this book, you should use discretion and common sense.

TABLE OF CONTENTS

THIS BOOK IS DEDICATED TO

. . all victims of arthritis, millions of you!

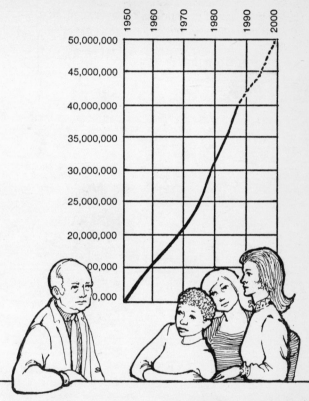

The total number of cases is climbing, tragically. More than 1,000,000 people are stricken annually. Throughout the United States, at this rate of increase, I forecast that *BY THE YEAR 2,000 THERE WILL BE 52,000,000 ARTHRITICS.*

"The doctor of the future will give no medicine, but will interest his patient in the case of the human frame, diet, and in the cause and prevention of disease."

Thomas A. Edison

Foreword

Dale Alexander is a questioning, openminded man who is very well-informed about health related sciences. He has devoted thirty-five years of his life to the study of the nutritional biochemistry of arthritis, and he has acquired some important knowledge of this painful and often disabling disorder.

During the course of his research, Alexander found convincing evidence that the onset of arthritis can often be directly related to a person's eating habits. He maintains that good nutrition—proper foods, consumed according to certain dietary rules—has helped thousands and can bring relief to millions of arthritic sufferers.

As a physician, it was necessary for me to carefully review Alexander's conclusions before I could recommend his course of treatment to any patients. To protect our patient's best interests, members of the medical profession must investigate any new approach to illness which promises better health before we adopt it or approve its use. We must be certain that it is safe and sufficiently effective to merit its use.

The time has come for arthritis sufferers and members of the healing professions to pay more attention to Dale Alexander's observations and conclusions.

In his first book, 35 years ago, he stated that arthritis sufferers could improve their condition by "lubricating" their arthritic joints, and that it was possible to accomplish this by following a correct diet. He advocated that arthritics should use a common sense approach in their selection of foods and beverages.

Throughout the years, he has continued to make observations that have convinced him that cod liver oil contains several substances which favorably affect the properties of the synovial fluid which lubricates the surfaces within joint cavities.

From the moment he reported his observations and conclusions, Alexander's method of treatment and nutritionally oriented concepts have been subjects of worldwide controversy. Some individual doctors and some spokesmen for different areas of the medical establishment immediately attacked his dietary program. They claimed that the normal consumption of foods in a "balanced diet has no role as a cause of arthritis. The preponderance of widely published medical research has been concentrated on the discovery and development of drugs to control or relieve arthritic pain. (Some of these drugs are potentially harmful—often associated with undesirable side effects.)

I have had experience treating patients suffering from allergies that definitely play an important role in "untreatable" or incurable conditions like multiple sclerosis, cerebral palsy, and arthritis. I am saddened by the opposition which other doctors have faced when they announced that vitamins could be helpful to relieve allergic-arthritis.

One of the pioneers in this field was William Kaufman, M.D., who was awarded the distinguished Tom Spies Memorial Award in Nutrition. He developed the effective use of niacinamide (Vitamin B-3) in the treatment of arthritis. Many of his patients experienced great improvement in their ability to move their arthritic joints because they had much less joint stiffness, discomfort and pain following Dr. Kaufman's program.

Let us keep in mind that the sincere and honest researcher who is pioneering a new course of action to alleviate the suffering and damage caused by arthritis or any disease is to be respected. For these dedicated efforts, he or she should be treated with courtesy and consideration.

Dale Alexander is an honorable man. He states that he has found a way to help the victims of arthritis "self-lubricate" their painful joints. In this book he presents all of his findings and he deserves the reader's careful attention as he reveals his sources of medical research. Can he substantiate his concepts with proven facts, by quoting recognized medical authorities? You, the reader, be the judge.

Dale Alexander has successfully used *nondrug nutritional therapy*. He wants to share his knowledge of this natural non-toxic and non-surgical approach with his fellow citizens. For millions of arthritics, I sincerely hope that his book will be an invaluable key to better health free of pain . . . a giant step toward achieving that goal.

Marshall Mandell, M.D.
Medical Director
New England Foundation for Allergic
and Environmental Diseases
Norwalk, Connecticut

August 1, 1984

CHAPTER I

Back Again . . . With More To Say

You and I have a mutual interest. Our goal is to resist and repel the painful misery of arthritis.

As I write this new book, my purpose is to bring you more facts and more answers——to help you conquer this illness. In these pages you will find the complete results of my work. Here are the key facts, important evidence I have gathered during the past 30 years.

My experiences——my worldwide travels since 1951——have convinced me that millions of arthritics can benefit from the ideas I shall now set forth in this manuscript.

When a man spends an entire lifetime studying just one disease, certainly he must learn some valuable information about that ailment. It is my hope that you will seriously consider the testimony which I now offer. I shall attempt to prove that arthritis is a constitutional disorder, not just an illness which causes aching, swollen joints.

Many of the Chapters, in this book, will also give witness to the fact that arthritis can be affected by good nutrition and proper diet. I will quote many physicians and scientists who believe as I do regarding certain dietary factors. You can now read about all the latest research, and evaluate it. Then, you can act . . . based on your own judgement and common sense.

I openly admit that my dietary program, designed to alleviate arthritis, is a theory. But I shall submit so many relevant facts, from so many sources, that you may agree with my logic and my conclusions.

Before you begin to read this manuscript, let's talk about credibility. You have the right to ask: "Who is this man, Dale Alexander? Where did he come from? What are his credentials, and is he qualified to discuss arthritis with any degree of authority?"

My reputation, as an author and lecturer, dates back to 1951. Yes, it was 33 years ago when the first volume of *Arthritis and Common Sense* was published. I never expected that the public response would be so overwhelming. I am deeply grateful that so many people saw merit in that book, and told their friends.

Now, more than 1,200,000 copies are in print, distributed throughout the world. I am humble, in awe of that total. Because I never intended to become an "author" . . . I just wanted to write a diary of facts about a remarkable experience which happened to my mother. She was a victim of crippling arthritis. By changing her diet, my mother recovered her health. Perhaps other people could benefit by reading her story. That was the simple intent of my first book.

Readers soon found that my dietary program was equally effective for them. The good news spread—and, quite by accident, suddenly I was catapulted into the role of being a "famous" author.

At first, the only way people heard about my book was by word-of-mouth. A relative or a friend was feeling better, thanks to some new method of eating.

Victims of arthritis, scattered in cities and towns across America, began reporting that their pain had receded. They were enjoying better health.

People, by the thousands, began talking about Dale Alexander. Was it possible that, somehow, he had found a partial solution to arthritic ailments?

The medical profession was quick to discount "the Alexander approach" . . . they announced it was too simple an answer. "Diet to combat arthritis? Nonsense!" Many doctors told their patients that the book was not responsible for improving health. "You are merely experiencing a period of spontaneous remission—the pain relief is only temporary."

But so many people reported long-lasting relief, there was no way to "bury" this encouraging news story. National magazines began writing articles . . . and, soon, I found myself being interviewed on the major television networks.

When I appeared on "The Arthur Godfrey Show" it drew an avalanche of mail. Millions of arthritics had questions to ask—and all the major TV programs invited me to respond. I went "on the air" with Mike Douglas, Merv Griffin, Johnny Carson.

So many people wrote letters—after my interview on "The Tonight Show"—the producers asked me to return for a second time. That night, David

Brenner was the guest host. We mixed in some humor, along with the serious suggestions about diet and nutrition.

I've always been just a quiet man, from a small town in Connecticut. So, those TV "talk shows" were exciting events for me. I was the "unknown author" who was swept into the spotlight, unawares.

The so-called "fame" which I have now acquired is not important. But it does serve one purpose. Now, I receive many more requests to lecture about arthritis . . . and that is my primary goal in life.

If I can teach about nutrition—speak before new audiences, throughout the world—I shall travel this earth to help arthritics.

MY QUEST FOR KNOWLEDGE . . . HOW IT ALL BEGAN

To learn everything possible about rheumatic illness, my early research was done in libraries. I studied medical literature, dozens of books. Many of them contained facts on arthritis, but the volumes were so ancient they had been forgotten and "lost" in the archives. With the help of librarians—in Hartford, Boston and New York—I traced the history of this illness, through the centuries.

I read about many remedies which had been tried in the past. But none of these "cures" had been truly successful, none of them had caused permanent relief from pain.

Time after time, as I was reading all these reports and scientific papers, the same two words kept appearing constantly. "Etiology unknown." No matter what type of arthritis was being discussed, the doctors would write that the real *cause* of this disease was still *unknown*.

After long months of searching in these medical libraries, however, I did find some clues. I saw a "pattern" of facts starting to develop.

It became obvious, to me, that arthritics were suffering from a lack of oil-bearing foods. Their bodies were "drying out" too often and too soon.

Dryness in the linings of their joints was the main problem to be solved. If I could find a way to *lubricate* tissues surrounding the joints, perhaps I could end my mother's pain-wracked ordeal.

Back in those days, before World War II, her ailment was simply called "rheumatism" . . . and she had a hopeless case. "Etiology unknown."

My first attempts to help her involved cod liver oil, and little else. But she did respond, remarkably well. Since then, I have expanded and improved my dietary program, based on added research and the wealth of information I have gathered from actual arthritics.

Later in this book, I shall offer an entire Chapter which gives a detailed description of *how* lubrication occurs within your body. I will discuss *digestion, absorption* and *assimilation*. These are the three keystones. What I say happens to the foods you digest does occur. My theory is physiologically possible . . . and I'll give you a pictorial map of where the oils travel.

PHASE TWO . . . MY EDUCATION AMONG ACTUAL ARTHRITICS

Most physicians must practice medicine in just one city or town. They open an office, and they can see only a few hundred patients per year. I enjoy a special advantage, because I have met thousands of arthritics, face-to-face, and I have listened to their specific questions about rheumatic ailments.

Everywhere I travel, the people who attend my lectures tell me about their personal experiences— how they have fought their own battles, what methods they have used as they try to "cure" their arthritis.

I have *learned* from all these encounters and discussions. It is possible that I have talked with more arthritics than any other man alive. All these lectures—spanning 30 years—have also allowed me to ask questions. When people told me about some new treatment they had tried, I would promptly investigate its powers to heal.

While preparing to write this book, I leafed through some of my scrapbooks. They are filled with newspaper clippings, a record of my travels. What marvelous memories! My early lecture tours took me to more than 95 cities throughout the United States.

I remember speaking in bookstores, on college campuses, in church basements, and in huge auditoriums. When it was announced that I would lecture in St. Petersburg, Florida, no hall was large enough. The event had to be held in a public park. That day, the total attendance was more than 6,000 people.

Another milestone was my first trip to Canada. The lecture took place, on campus, at the University of British Columbia.

Jet aircraft makes any journey possible. I flew to South Africa . . . traveled to Johannesburg. There, I spoke before 90 doctors, residents and interns at the University of Witwatersand.

Next, came invitations to lecture in Australia. I accepted immediately, and took off for Melbourne.

The friendly people, throughout Australia, gave me a warm welcome. They were eager to hear my views about arthritis—because this disease has swept across that continent, worsening every year. I was questioned closely, at the University of Sydney. That nation also broadcasts an Australian edition of "Meet The Press"—and I appeared on that program. The telecast became an excellent debate, as I argued in behalf of better nutrition.

Other clippings, pasted in my scrapbook, describe my repeated lectures in England, Ireland and Wales. I have flown to London three separate times—in order to meet with readers of my book. I toured the British Isles including Scotland, lecturing in a dozen different cities.

Arthritis has now invaded every nation, around the world. This harrowing illness has spread across oceans—to every outpost of civilization. It has even struck people who live on islands in the South Seas.

I went to New Zealand, because arthritics there needed help. In that country, I lectured in Dunedin, at the Otago Medical School.

Incidentally, a purported "cure" for arthritis has surfaced in New Zealand. I have checked it out, and I'll report my findings in Chapter III of this book. The treatment is being developed by a marine pharmacologist. Experiments indicate that shellfish may contain therapeutic substances. Being tested are mussels, grown in the waters near Auckland, New Zealand.

As I mention these travels of mine, I am not just reminiscing. There's a point to be made. I want you to know the extent of my past education.

I circle the globe, on a constant quest for the truth about arthritis. I talk with surgeons, and pathologists, and biochemists. I visit laboratories and clinics, attend conferences and seminars.

Yes, I am self-educated. And I'm proud of it!

The most significant fact is that I have met with thousands of people who *had* arthritis. They experienced this painful affliction, personally. Bless them all! They gave me their knowledge, to share with you.

So, I shall write this book, hoping to shed some light on a difficult topic. There's a certain clipping, in my scrapbook, which describes my one goal in life. The editors of *Healthview Newsletter* interviewed me, and here's what they wrote:

Dale Alexander is a layman who became interested in arthritis back in the late 1920's, when his mother was stricken with the disease.

"I saw her suffer," he says, "for 10 long years. I know the damage arthritis can do to a person and to her family.

"Over the years, her condition gradually deteriorated. The swelling increased. Her knees began to give out. Her fingers became so stiff she could barely open or close her hands. The pain was so constant and intense you could hardly say she was living any more—she was barely existing.

"I felt heartbroken to see her suffering—and frustrated because there was nothing I could do about it. It was so maddening that one day something snapped inside of me. I had to do something, anything, to help her. I couldn't watch her suffering any more. From that moment on, I've devoted my life to helping my mother—and all arthritic sufferers like her."

CHAPTER II

A Typical Interview . . . Probing My Views

Journalists—the working press—are not admired when they ask hard-hitting questions. Any author who agrees to an interview should certainly expect to be interrogated closely.

I welcome such sessions . . . where the newspapermen or magazine writers demand honest answers. They want confirmation, added facts, to support every statement you make. That's fine, the way it should be.

For the most part, the interviewers I have faced have been fair-minded and friendly. But, once in awhile, I encounter a writer who is anti-nutrition and says so from the start.

Let me give you an example of how it feels to be interviewed "in depth" . . . when the questions are tough, and nobody pulls any punches.

One reason I respect *Healthview Newsletter*— see clipping page 13—is the caliber of their editors. They search hard for news, so they compiled a list of far-reaching questions. "Find out what makes Alexander tick. Put him through the mill."

For this special interview, I traveled to them. Ready to meet, I arrived at their editorial offices, in

Charlottesville, Virginia. They were skeptical, I guess. They began by asking a "loaded" question . . .

HEALTHVIEW NEWSLETTER: Obviously, you had a good measure of success with your mother, or you wouldn't have published your book. How did you, as a layman, with no medical background at all, come to develop a successful program where thousands of doctors have failed?

ALEXANDER: I started off by reading everything about arthritis I could get my hands on. I began to haunt the medical libraries. At first, I couldn't find anything of value. Everything I came across my mother had already tried—heat, ointments (you can't imagine how many different kinds), drugs, exercises. They had even extracted her teeth—a popular treatment at the time. But none of these had given her more than mild, temporary relief—so I knew I had to go further.

HEALTHVIEW NEWSLETTER: What did you do?

ALEXANDER: I kept going. My research went in two directions—interestingly enough they were opposite.

On the one hand, I pursued all the latest medical findings and current research. On the other hand, I started digging into the past, into forgotten "remedies" and "folk cures".

Needless to say, the great bulk of the material was worthless. But, in an old medical book, published in 1855, I came upon one old-time folk remedy that was to prove to be the lost "key" to solving the problems of arthritis.

The book was by a medical doctor, a Dr. L. J.

deJong, who had tested it in his daily practice. He had found that it worked better than anything else he had ever heard of.

The doctor had no idea of why it worked, but the more I thought about it, the more sense it made to me. It seemed to fit the facts about arthritis—which we'll get into later. But back then, what was very important to me was that the remedy was completely safe. It could do only good: at worst my mother's condition would be unchanged. So I spoke with her about it. She decided to give it a fair try.

HEALTHVIEW NEWSLETTER: What happened?

ALEXANDER: At first, nothing.

Then, after 10 weeks, the first in a series of curious changes came over her. Her hair, which had been lifeless and dry, began to recover its lustre and sheen.

During the twelfth week, another change occurred. Her skin, always very dry, became soft and supple.

Next, she discovered a new sensation in her ears. She found that, for the first time in years, she was developing ear wax—which is normal in a healthy person.

The last, and most notable change, was the one we had been seeking all along—relief from her arthritic condition. In the middle of the fifth month—that's quite some time—it happened. Her fingers and arms began to lose their swelling and stiffness. The pain began to recede. Next, her knees began to feel better, and finally her back.

Once the first sign of improvement had begun, the whole process moved quite rapidly. Before long there was pain-free motion! After so many years of suffering, her long ordeal was over.

We were so happy, we cried.

HEALTHVIEW NEWSLETTER: What was that remedy you gave her?

ALEXANDER: Oddly enough, it was plain old cod liver oil. It sounds like an unlikely solution, doesn't it? But you ought to see what it can do for arthritis.

What cod liver oil does is to increase the quality of the joint fluid. You see, the basic cause of arthritis is that the lubricating fluid in the joints gets too thin. It doesn't lubricate properly. So, naturally, your joints become stiff and difficult to move.

When human joints lack the proper lubricating fluid, the various parts of the joint—the cartilage, the joint lining, the bony parts—begin to rub and grind against one another. There's friction, then stiffness, then irritation, and then finally inflammation. That's just what the word arthritis means: inflammation of the joints. "Arth" means joint and "itis" means inflammation.

Incidentally, it doesn't matter what kind of arthritis you have, they all respond to cod liver oil. The reason for this is that all arthritis—regardless of the symptoms—has the same basic cause: poorly lubricated joints. It's just that each person reacts differently.

For example, if friction causes the cartilage to

wear away, we call it osteoarthritis. If it's the joint lining that suffers, it's rheumatoid arthritis. No matter what the symptoms, cod liver oil will help.

HEALTHVIEW NEWSLETTER: That's an interesting theory. Do you have any evidence to back it up?

ALEXANDER: I certainly do. I didn't just read a few articles on cod liver oil, and run out and publish a book. I knew I had a big responsibility——both to the public and to the medical profession.

I knew I was definitely on to something, but I realized I had to back up my theories with solid, indisputable evidence. Otherwise, why should anyone pay attention to me.

As soon as my mother was back on her feet, I returned to the medical libraries to pick up where I had left off.

I found a report in Dr. Pemberton's book, *The Medical Management of Arthritis,* which showed that normal people have joint fluid that's over 15 times as thick and viscous as the fluid in arthritic joints. What a difference! It shows the tremendous variation in joint fluid between a healthy person and an arthritic.

I learned that the joint linings can accept nutritional oils directly from the bloodstream. I also learned that cartilage——the tissue next to the bone——could absorb these oils from the lining, through osmosis.

(*EDITOR'S NOTE:* In this interview, the questions by *Healthview Newsletter* have been quoted exactly word for word. The answers, given by Alexander, have been edited slightly . . . primarily to condense his replies and conserve space in this book.)

HEALTHVIEW NEWSLETTER: Has cod liver oil ever been tested by the medical profession?

ALEXANDER: Many times. Medical literature is full of accounts of its use as a folk remedy two hundred years back in the treatment of arthritis.

More recently, in 1920, to be precise, cod liver oil was tested and approved by Dr. Ralph Pemberton of the University of Pennsylvania. He was one of the leading rheumatologists of all time. The highest honor a rheumatologist can receive today is to be called upon to give the annual Pemberton Lecture on Rheumatology. That gives you an idea of the esteem in which Dr. Pemberton is held.

Dr. Pemberton tested cod liver oil on hundreds of arthritic patients. He reported his findings in his report entitled, *Studies on Arthritis in the Army Based on Four Hundred Cases,* which appeared in the *Archives of Internal Medicine* (March, 1920.).

After thorough testing, Dr. Pemberton concluded that cod liver oil was effective in eliminating the pain, stiffness and swelling of chronic arthritis. This is quite an endorsement, coming from a man like Dr. Pemberton.

I know the theory works, because over the years, I've received thousands of letters from people throughout America—and later around the world—who have tried cod liver oil.

For instance, I received a letter from a woman in St. Petersburg, Florida. Let me read it to you . . . She said:

"Dear Dale Alexander,

Twenty-five years ago, I was unable to walk. Every joint in my body was aching. My husband had to carry me up the stairs. I was unable to walk. My doctors told me I would eventually have to be in a wheelchair.

"I read your book and took cod liver oil. In one month, I was able to walk and work. The pain was gone. Now and then I go off the cod liver oil and the pain comes back. So, I go back to it and I am alright again, thank God. If it were not for your book, I would today be a complete invalid."

(*AUTHOR'S COMMENT:* I showed that letter, and others like it, to the editors who were interviewing me. They saw written proof that cod liver oil is a viable weapon against arthritis. People write to me all the time—sincere, thankful letters—and they inspire me to continue my research work.)

I never resent it when journalists express some doubt about my dietary theories. They have a right to demand medical confirmation and supporting facts. The writers are being vigilant, protecting their readers.

You may have noticed that this interview—with *Healthview Newsletter*—contained repeated questions which were asked with a tone of skepticism. They were "grilling" me. In fact, at the end, this was their very last query:

"What does the medical profession think of your program?"

I replied, quite frankly, that some doctors are still attacking my nutritional claims. But attitudes are changing, in my favor. This was my final answer:

ALEXANDER: I think it's only a matter of time before the medical profession will turn to diet as a real "cure" for arthritis. It happened with insulin. Not too many years ago, doctors relied on insulin to control diabetes. Now, they recognize diet as an accepted and preferred method of treatment. I predict the same thing will happen with arthritis.

The future outlook is encouraging. For readers of this book, I shall list the most beneficial foods. But, first, here are *all the facts* on cod liver oil . . .

WHERE ARTHRITIS ATTACKS
MOST FREQUENTLY

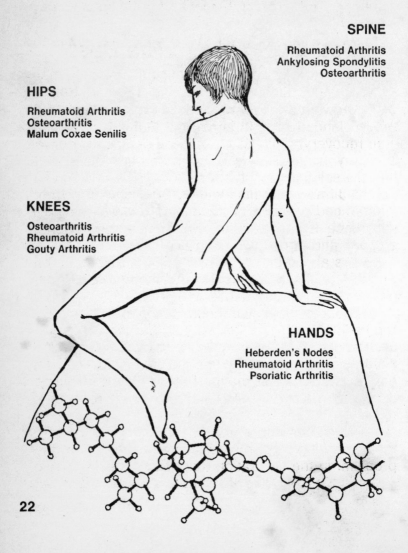

SPINE

Rheumatoid Arthritis
Ankylosing Spondylitis
Osteoarthritis

HIPS

Rheumatoid Arthritis
Osteoarthritis
Malum Coxae Senilis

KNEES

Osteoarthritis
Rheumatoid Arthritis
Gouty Arthritis

HANDS

Heberden's Nodes
Rheumatoid Arthritis
Psoriatic Arthritis

22

CHAPTER III

Cod Liver Oil . . . The Best Solution

Knowing the correct foods to eat, and having a truly balanced diet, is important. But the speed of your recovery will definitely depend on cod liver oil. It can be your greatest ally. As an anti-arthritic agent, this oily solution has no equal!

Until now, like most people, you have probably ignored cod liver oil. You have tried to forget the fishy substance. It was something your mother poured into a spoon and forced you to swallow.

"As a medication, this oil doesn't belong in the Space Age. It's an old-fashioned remedy. Used by my grandmother, for her aches and pains."

I hear remarks like these, almost every day. By reputation, cod liver oil is just an ancient cure-all. People sometimes smile, bemused, when I recommend they try it. So, now, I intend to write an entire chapter on this matter. Perhaps if you know the complete history of cod liver oil, you'll respect it more.

No matter where arthritis strikes in your body, the lubricating properties of this oil can alleviate the problem. In the Illustration (opposite page) we could show only a few types of arthritis. It's a grim fact, but doctors can now diagnose more than 100 ailments as being some form of "arthritic" disease.

Your first step, on the road to recovery, is to learn what "type" of arthritis is ruining your life. Know your enemy. With 100 different "varieties" to choose from, only a qualified physician or a trained rheumatologist can determine the exact nature of your illness.

I have always recommended that any person who is ill should consult a doctor——for a complete physical examination. Describe your arthritic symptoms to him, ask him all the questions you can concerning the form of treatment he proposes. (If you wish, show him this book. See what he thinks about cod liver oil.)

If your doctor wants to "study up on the subject"——before rendering his verdict——you might suggest that he read a certain medical paper. The special report was written by a physician from the Department of Pediatrics, Yale University School of Medicine. The title is: *The History of Cod Liver Oil as a Remedy*.

I might add, most respectfully, that the author was a woman. A lady doctor. Her research work was monumental. She traced the use of cod liver oil, and discovered it has been effective as a medicine for hundreds of years. I extend my congratulations to her——to Ruth Guy, M.D.——for a job well done (see page 272).

HISTORIC HIGHLIGHTS . . . DOWN THROUGH THE CENTURIES

America was fighting a war in 1776, and there's no record that George Washington took cod liver oil on any regular basis. But, in England, physicians were already prescribing the oil for chronic rheumatism. In 1771 it was entered in the British Pharmacopaeia.

Old documents state that patients were given cod liver oil at the Manchester Infirmary . . . so frequently that the institution used "near a hogshead annually".

In 1807, a Dr. Bardsley of that same Infirmary gave his findings on cod liver oil. He reported: "It has operated in a manner so decidedly beneficial as to excite astonishment."

In 1910, according to Dr. Guy, an expert named Rosenstern made a very valid statement. He wrote: "Cod liver oil is in the forefront of children's remedies. For long it has been struggling against the skepticism of exact science." (editor's underlining)

For anyone who might still be skeptical, I have a true story to tell. Let me recall an historic event which happened during World War II . . .

When Hitler had London under seige, the British government feared that food supplies would be cut off—endangering the health of babies and toddlers. So they enacted a law to provide all children with a "ration" of two key products. Throughout the war, these two crucial items were supplied to families.

What were the two chosen products, considered so vital? Orange juice and cod liver oil.

Today, scientific laboratories in the United States have the capability to analyze oil-bearing foods. I must report, however, that the most extensive research work on cod liver oil has been carried out by British workers in the clinics and hospitals of Europe.

They have established the importance of certain polyunsaturated fatty acids—including EPA and DHA—which are known to be present in cod liver oil.

Would you like to read my detailed description of their highly technical experiments? I could explain that EPA is eicosapentaenoic acid . . . and DHA is docosahexaenoic acid. But I believe that their favorable affect, in our fight against arthritis, ought to be stated in very simple terms. I shall try to do so, later in this book, when I discuss "osmosis" and how your body can *absorb* beneficial oils.

For now, just let me emphasize that the world of science is actively studying cod liver oil. *Since 1978* there has been more major research published on this subject than for the previous 50 years!

THE RUSSIANS ARE COMING!

They have gone into battle. The Soviet Union is our ally, this time. In the war against arthritis.

Russian scientists have already conducted

some valuable experiments . . . a series of medical tests which may lead to a cure for rheumatic illness.

Arthritis is an affliction which transcends all political boundaries. If the Soviets can be the first to discover an effective remedy, their success will be deserved. Because they have been quietly working on the problem for at least three decades.

I recently obtained a special report, translated from Russian, concerning research work which was done by I. I. Khvorostukhin from the Stanilslausk Medical Institute.

After studying this material I was amazed. The report revealed that the Russians were experimenting with *cod liver oil* . . . as far back as 1961!

What the Russian scientists tried to prove was this: ''Can damaged joint cartilage repair itself and be regenerated?''

If victims of arthritis could be given the gift of healthy cartilage, these laboratory tests would be of historic importance.

Unfortunately, the Russians employed a technique which I deplore. They performed operations on 22 dogs. Each animal was inflicted with bone cartilage injuries in both knee joints.

(I condemn most experiments using animals. See Chapter XIV, where I offer my humane opinions.)

Next, the Russians *injected* cod liver oil——hoping to stimulate the regeneration of cartilage. I have never proposed injecting the oil in animals or humans.

For nearly six months, the dogs were observed and microscopic studies were made. Some regeneration of cartilage was reported. But, for better results, they should change the testing procedures. Next time, experiment with human beings . . . and let them take cod liver oil *orally*.

WE TRAVEL ON . . . FROM MOSCOW TO THE SOUTH PACIFIC

For a vacation, to relax in the sun, let's visit the tropical islands near New Zealand. Last time I was there, I had no time to enjoy life. The people of New Zealand kept me busy answering questions about arthritis. They are fighting to banish this illness.

As an example of their efforts, let me tell you a fish story. A shellfish story. This is the saga of New Zealand Green-Lipped Mussels . . .

A scientist named John E. Croft has derived an extract from mussels. The product is taken orally, and some arthritics have reported therapeutic results.

It is interesting to note that, once again, the remedy is related to marine life. I say codfish can yield the necessary oils. He proclaims that mussels hold the answer.

Experiments continue in New Zealand—with mussels being grown in aquatic farms. I am not surprised by these developments. In the past, chemists have analyzed shark oil, whale oil, and dozens of alternatives. None can match the advantages of cod liver oil.

John Croft has a book of his own. The title—

Natural Relief from Arthritis—states a commendable goal. I agree with him on one major point. There is great truth in his concluding comments. He wrote:

"So far, using substances found on land, we have not been successful in finding a cure for diseases like cancer, leukemia and multiple sclerosis. The treatments which remedy these and other serious disorders may very well be awaiting discovery in a very obvious place—the ocean."

End quote. A perfect summary. No wonder I am such a staunch advocate of cod liver oil.

CHAPTER IV

Absorb The Oils . . . It Can Be Done!

From the very start I have always maintained that certain oils—contained in certain foods—can be beneficial to the linings of your joints.

I've been saying this for 30 years. The human body is capable of digesting and absorbing oils . . . it can *self-lubricate* arthritic joints.

By eliminating dryness, your joints can move more easily, pain recedes, and better health is the happy reward.

This theory of "lubrication" which I advanced was immediately challenged by some segments of the medical profession. The critics, doctors among them, made statements like these:

"The dietary plan proposed by Alexander is too simple an answer. He's a layman, so he probably knows very little about basic physiology."

Apparently they would prefer that I use more "medical language" and more technical terms. Whenever I discuss human anatomy or digestive organs, I guess they want me to "sound" like a doctor. Why? Just to prove I have education and knowledge on these topics?

My first responsibility is to you, the reader. I will

not subject you to a complicated vocabulary. My message can be told in clear, understandable words. The picture below can explain it all. Just turn this page . . .

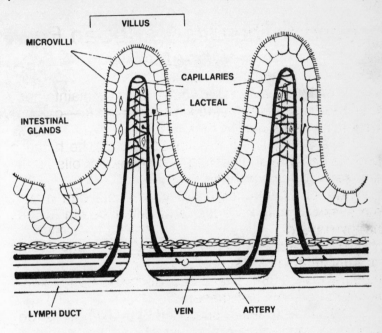

HOW AND WHERE OILS ARE ABSORBED. . .
TO "LUBRICATE" AGAINST ARTHRITIS
(Cross-Section View of Your Intestinal Wall)

Imagine that you are looking at the interior of your small intestine . . . less than one inch of it is shown in the illustration on previous page.

Inside your gastro-intestinal tract are thousands of tiny projections, each called a *villus.* The artist has drawn just *two* of them—those two "hilly" objects seen in the diagram. Now, look closely at the needle-like area (shaded in grey) inside the capillaries. These are "lacteals" and *they are the conduits which can help carry the proper dietary oils to arthritic joints.* Your primary goal should be to deliver Vitamin D_3 oil to the lacteals.

This route I am describing is using systemic circulation to carry oil globules, microscopically small, toward the lining of your joints.

For example, when the cod liver oil mixture which I recommend is taken on an empty stomach, it is carried by the lacteals until it is later absorbed or assimilated within the body.

These lymph vessels (the lacteals) then transport the oil to a major oil collecting "depot" within your system known as the cisterna chyli. Then it is picked up by the thoracic duct—and the cod liver oil is delivered into the lymphatic system. It is piped into the main bloodstream as minute chylomicrons.

By taking cod liver oil you are "loading" the chylomicrons with Vitamin D, Vitamin A, and Vitamin F. You are using systemic circulation to carry these oil-soluble vitamins and essential fatty acids to the locations in your body where they are needed most.

In effect, when you by-pass the greedy liver in

this manner, you can deliver Vitamin D *intact* to the lining of the joints!

This process of absorbing the oils works best when you don't drink water with your meals. If you omit water, I maintain that your digestive system can deliver approximately 90% of the Vitamin D oil to your lacteals. The capillaries will capture the remaining 10%. But, healthwise, you're way ahead.

To help explain "digestion" and "assimilation"—in simple terms, easy to understand—there's another drawing you should study. Please turn to Page 296. Consult that Illustration, and learn more facts.

I insist that oil can "travel" to the linings of your joints. Some doctors have questioned this fact. Which baffles me, because this is not just my theory. It is not something I invented. Many distinguished scientists did the initial research. They deserve full credit for exploring this type of lipid metabolism.

We are discussing how oil is metabolized—how it is absorbed by your body. Medical literature has been publishing learned articles on this topic for the past 40 years!

SOURCE MATERIAL . . . PROOF ABOUT "ABSORBING" OILS

The real pioneer in this field of lipid (oil) metabolism is Dr. A.C. Frazer. Way back in 1945, he reported the results of his research in *The Journal of Physiology*.

Doctor Frazer conducted tests which showed how hydrolyzed oils can be drawn primarily into the lymphatic system of your body. Instead of traveling the portal route—to your liver—these large chain fatty acids would be absorbed by the lymph ducts.

In my first book, 33 years ago, I mentioned Doctor Frazer's work. I also commended Dr. Abraham White, the noted biochemist at Yale University. He wrote a revealing chapter on this subject. It appeared in a book entitled *Diseases of the Metabolism.* That volume was published in 1947.

I repeat, this theory is not new . . . and it is not revolutionary.

Both of these men inspired my thinking . . . set me off on a search for more answers.

For example, one factor which I learned from Dr. Frazer was the importance of using hydrolyzed oil. Break down the oil globules—emulsify them, so they can travel through your digestive system more easily. That's why I recommend that you mix cod liver oil with orange juice or milk. Shake it well, to make the emulsification more complete.

As the years went by, the evidence mounted. In 1959, Dr. Samuel Gurin contributed his findings to the fourth edition of *Diseases of the Metabolism.* He told how investigations were conducted concerning the route of transport of saturated acids with different chain lengths.

(Let me clarify what "chain length" means. It is

simply a term that biochemists use to describe the carbon content in various fatty acids. For instance, cod liver oil is considered to be "long chain"— because it contains 22 atoms of carbon per molecule. Butter and eggs are in the "short chain" category, with only about 4 carbon atoms in their molecular structure.)

Doctor Gurin cited research work which suggested that the shorter chain acids may be transported largely by way of the portal circulation. In other words, through the liver!

But, to quote Dr. Gurin: "It would appear, therefore, that the long-chain saturated and unsaturated acids <u>are</u> <u>preferentially</u> <u>transported</u> <u>by</u> <u>way</u> <u>of</u> <u>the</u> <u>lymphatics</u>."

The underlining is mine, for emphasis. He is stating, as I have for years, the same basic fact: Oils *can travel* through your body via lymph ducts.

When I learned it was possible to "direct" the flow of oils to various parts of one's body that *fact* became the cornerstone for my future research.

At that time—in the early 1940's—there was one major question still unresolved. Some way, I had to determine *which oil* would be most beneficial for arthritics.

By pouring over medical journals, for weeks on end, I discovered repeated references to cod liver oil. You already know, from Chapter III, how medical history favored this oil. It was the logical choice.

Dietary *common sense* was all I prescribed in my original book. My nutritional findings are not based on some mysterious formula. Any pre-med student who is taught basic physiology will realize how metabolism works. Even so, some doctors still act surprised when my dietary program reduces pain.

The key element—to be metabolized by your body—is cod liver oil. Mainly because this substance contains Vitamin D_3 for the lubrication process. Not long ago, I decided to obtain a "picture" of Vitamin D_3. I went to a computer scientist, at UCLA, and asked for his help. For the whole story, see the next page . . .

If you are ready to try a nutritional approach, study mine. Compare my plan with other diets . . . a rash of them are being announced on newsstands.

Every few weeks, another national magazine will suddenly feature a major story on what happens when arthritics seek relief through some form of diet. I'll comment, shortly, about which publishers to trust.

WHAT DOES "VITAMIN D" LOOK LIKE?

At several points throughout this book you may have noticed an odd-shaped drawing—with many prongs and tiny circles, tied together in a futuristic design.

That same piece of artwork is repeated on quite a few pages. Why? Because it is a true "portrait" of Vitamin D_3—one of the most valuable elements found in cod liver oil.

As I was writing this book, I began to wonder if modern technology could "draw" an accurate symbol of this health-rich substance.

So, I traveled to the Chemistry Department at the University of California in Los Angeles. There, I met with Dr. Charles E. Strouse. He is widely respected, known for the research work he performs in the X-ray Crystallography Laboratory at UCLA.

Dr. Strouse determined the atomic coordinates of this vitamin. Information was fed into a huge Digital computer. Contact was made with a scientific Data Bank—in Cambridge, England. Some answers were transmitted from this source in Great Britain.

The computer then drew every molecule . . . and the "print-out" it delivered was quite remarkable. Next, I asked an artist to copy the computer drawing exactly. If you turn to the very front of this book, for the first time you can *see* Vitamin D_3.

"PREVENTION" MAGAZINE . . . PUBLISHING THE TRUTH!

Arthritis was the subject of a five-page article in *Prevention* Magazine not long ago. I congratulate the editors and staff of that publication for a superb job of reporting.

Everyone afflicted with arthritis could relate to what the writer said. He gave an honest, up-to-date description of the latest methods which arthritics are using to gain relief.

I was so favorably impressed, I telephoned the magazine. My purpose was to commend the staff . . . they did some outstanding research work, compiling background facts for the article.

An editorial decision was made at *Prevention* which caused the magazine to conduct an entire project on arthritis. Robert Rodale, the Editor, writes a monthly column. In one edition, he invited his loyal readers who had arthritis to send him letters. He asked for a progress report on what steps they were taking to fight the disease.

The mail response was immediate. Overwhelming! Hundreds of letters poured into *Prevention* offices. Some were tragic, as arthritics told their own stories of pain and anguish.

But many of the letters offered hope, talked of remedies which had worked successfully. People wanted to share their experiences, in order to help arthritics everywhere. So, Editor Rodale wrote a special column based on his incoming mail. (I shall quote from that remarkable column, later in this chapter.)

I am especially pleased that this authentic survey was conducted, and by this unique publication, because I have watched the growth of *Prevention* since it was founded back in 1949. When it was still a small magazine, I was lecturing in Allentown, Pennsylvania. Jerome Rodale invited me to his home, to have dinner. We sat around and talked about his dreams to publish an *important* magazine . . . to *serve* the health-conscious public.

Even then, in 1952, in regard to arthritis I was a

proponent for proper diet and cod liver oil. I told
Jerome Rodale about my theories. On many subjects,
he and I were of the same mind. We believed that
people should have civil liberty . . . freedom of choice
in matters of personal health, as long as such choices
do not infringe upon the liberties of others.

Now, of course, *Prevention* has grown to become America's leading health magazine. More than
3,000,000 copies are published every month. Robert
Rodale has become Editor——and he often states cou-
rageous views on many health topics. He is carrying
on the tradition of his late father.

Here is a current example of editorial bravery.
Robert Rodale devoted his entire column to various
methods whereby his readers who suffer from
arthritis *can* achieve *Alternate Pain Relief.* He wrote:

> "Perhaps some day no one will be surprised or
> put off by anecdotal information. And maybe no one
> will raise an eyebrow when they hear of the alterna-
> tive arthritis therapies you detail in your letters. Mas-
> sages, hot baths or showers, ice packs, heating pads,
> positive visualization (imagining a reduction in pain),
> alfalfa tablets, acupuncture——many of you swear by
> these and others. Some are known painkillers, others
> make good physiological sense though there's little
> or no research yet to confirm them, and a few are just
> plain mysterious. They all, however, fall under the
> grand principle that so many arthritis victims have
> come to respect: If it relieves the hurt, it's good medi-
> cine.
>
> "One alternative remedy that wears that label
> more than most is cod-liver oil. In our informal poll it
> drew an extraordinary amount of praise, and I think I

know why. A while back some researchers at Brusch Medical Center in Cambridge, Massachusetts, gave daily doses of the supplement to nearly a hundred arthritics (some suffering from osteoarthritis, others from rheumatoid arthritis, others with gout). The result was a major improvement in 93 percent of the patients. They had less fatigue, less swelling and better mobility. And these people had failed just about every conventional arthritis treatment you can name.

"Well, many of you heard about the study, gave the remedy a try and filed your report with our arthritis survey. Here's a typical assessment of cod-liver oil's effect on arthritis symptoms: *'My osteoarthritis frightened me most when it began to spread. First it struck my hands, then one knee stiffened, then the other. I couldn't sit unless my right leg was extended and supported. Then suddenly my left knee became much more inflamed and tender. I feared that I was losing my ability to walk. But about that time I heard about cod-liver oil for arthritis. So I started taking a tablespoon of it just before bedtime, and very quickly my most painful symptoms eased up. Now I can actually do my gardening again.'*

* *AUTHOR'S NOTE:* That letter, from a reader of *Prevention* Magazine who lives in Rochester, New York, is very similar to the mail I receive from people who have studied my previous book. After they add cod liver oil to their daily diet, they report definite results.

I would also like to make one other observation, just as an historic footnote. This magazine article, quoted above, mentions the research work performed at the Brusch Medical Center. I am pleased to say that it was I who initiated that series of tests years ago. I requested that clinical evaluation of my theories . . . the patients followed my dietary rules and were given cod liver oil. Some members of the medical profession have discounted and disparaged the Brusch experiments, but I still maintain that it was a valuable research project.

By changing their sequence of eating, some of those patients had a beneficial drop in their cholesterol levels—by as much as 30%. Also, abnormal levels of blood sugar dropped to normal ranges.

"Maybe the oil's secret is its high content of vitamin D, the nutrient that helps keep your body using its calcium. Or maybe the active ingredient is some unknown substance that enhances joint lubrication. Whatever the biochemistry is, you can be sure that to those in pain, relief itself counts far more than its cause.

"And I suspect that in the long run, the specific remedy isn't nearly as important as the attitudes that engender it. The courage to never give any ground to the pain, the good sense to stay open to healing options—this is the right stuff. And plenty of you have it."

To those inspiring statements by the Editor of *Prevention* Magazine, I can only add one word: "Amen!"

DOCTORS DENOUNCE DIET . . . THEY OFFER "ASPIRIN" INSTEAD!

They are still doing it, almost every physician in practice today. To treat arthritis, they usually prescribe some pain-killer, available at your local pharmacy.

Drugs are the most popular antidote. As students in medical school, the fledgling doctors were taught to rely on pharmaceutical *products.* Courses were given on which "pills" were best. They learned about all the medicants being manufactured—one for every disease in the book!

Unfortunately, in most cases, they had a great "gap" in their education. Very few classes were held on *Nutrition*.

They graduated, with their M.D. degrees. But most members of the medical profession still have a "blind spot" concerning proper diet.

However, let's be fair. Let's consider "drugs" . . . and evaluate some actual products, old and new, which have been prescribed for arthritics.

To cover this topic, truthfully, I shall now write an entire Chapter about drugs. Read on. . .

CHAPTER V

Drugs To Relieve Arthritis . . . Just A Dream?

Throughout history real doctors and witch doctors have been sticking needles into people, using drugs to "cure" arthritis.

Sometimes their use of injections has been based on nothing more than wishful thinking. The ancient Chinese, for example, were treated with a golden needle. If the joints in their shoulders ached, they would show their doctor the exact spot. Then, he "stuck" the patient with a needle—containing no serum or vaccine—just the needle! (This may have been the prelude to the healing art now known as acupuncture.)

In the 16th Century, some medicine men in France began to prescribe "gold salts" to relieve arthritic pains. Porterius, a French physician, started using colloidal gold compounds—and certain doctors still recommend this metallic substance to this very day.

The point I am making is that *no injection* has yet been discovered which can stop the worldwide spread of arthritis. Drugs have not prevented the tragic growth of this disease. *No pills* can conquer arthritis . . . the pharmaceutical companies are still searching for the answer.

43

There are too many types of arthritic ailments—too many categories of pain—for any one drug to be totally effective.

I do not deny that medical science has *tried* to find a potent product for drug therapy. Many readers of this book are probably ingesting pills or taking injections—because someone told them they might help to some degree.

For about ten years, from 1950 to 1960, one of the most popular solutions was ACTH. Injections of Adrenal Cortical Trophic Hormone were touted to high heaven. More recently, doctors have needled their patients with penicillamine or prednisolone.

The favorites, for oral consumption, now include everything from aspirin, to colchicine for gouty arthritis, to phenylbutazone for rheumatoid illness.

WHAT HAPPENED TO CORTISONE?

Synthetic cortisone, taken orally or by injection, has started to fade from the limelight . . . it has lost its appeal among many doctors and patients.

The decline began about 1965. By then, too many victims of arthritis were reporting harmful side effects from using test-tube cortisone. While the drug did bring temporary pain relief to some people, this gain was often nullified when they developed several other annoying afflictions.

Patients learned that synthetic cortisone had a "ballooning" affect on their faces. In addition to be-

ARTHRITIS IS A CONSTITUTIONAL DISORDER
NOT LIMITED TO YOUR JOINTS

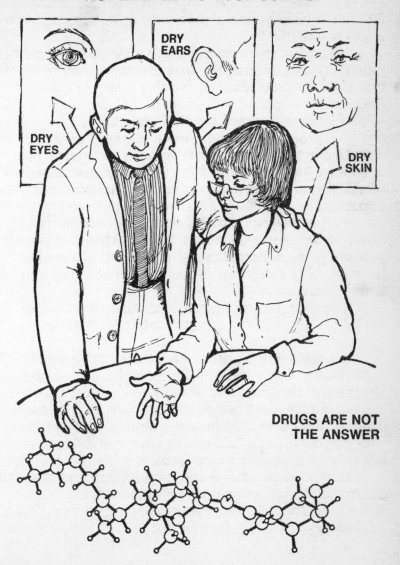

coming "moon faced" some people began to grow hair in the wrong places—like women suddenly finding they had mustaches.

Worse, many women who were in their menopausal stage discovered that the cortisone drug would cause accentuated flushing and high blood pressure.

If you pick up a copy of my first book, you will find that I spend two full pages warning everyone about the potential danger of synthetic cortisone. I am not clairvoyant. But, even then, thirty-five years ago, I was urging arthritics to manufacture their own natural cortisone.

Yes, within your body, right now, *cortisone* is being secreted from the outer bark or layers of your adrenal glands. And this natural cortisone is of a higher quality than any concocted version you can find in a pharmacy.

The secret is, of course, to stimulate your adrenal glands. Activate the adrenals, so they create more and better cortisone.

It has been proven that the adrenals will respond to a steroid, like Vitamin D. Use cod liver oil as the stimulator. Mix the oil with orange juice, as described in this book. If you emulsify the cod liver oil, you can send oil bubbles containing the nutritive Vitamin D to your adrenal glands. Simple and safe. You will not experience any harmful side effects.

Cortisone, made the natural way, has a heavier quality. It is more "sticky" and may increase the consistency of the collagen in your body.

(Collagen is that glue-like protein substance which supports bone, cartilage, ligaments, tendons and other connective tissues.)

To sum it up, I am in favor of cortisone, if you allow Nature to make it for you. When you create it internally you add viscosity to your collagen—so that *oils will be held in place near your joints.*

In a way, what we are talking about in this Chapter is drug abuse. Too many drugs, prescribed for arthritics, are causing abusive side effects, harmful to your body. Dr. Robert Mendelsohn cited a sad example . . . so typical and truthful that I have quoted his remarks. (See page 207 of this book.)

A DRUG WORTH MENTIONING . . . DMSO

It may be the most talked about drug in the world today. A full-scale controversy is raging, and I certainly intend to offer my opinions on the value of DMSO.

DIMETHYL SULFOXIDE (which the public knows as DMSO) has already survived intense criticism, and has earned our serious consideration as a weapon against arthritis.

DMSO may be the only drug to receive favorable mention in this entire book. I am inclined to admit that this natural product does bring temporary relief for *some types* of arthritis. I'll be more specific in just a moment. But, first, let's examine the pro and con arguments which have made DMSO hard to purchase anywhere in the United States.

Arthritics are running off to Mexico, paying "rip-off" prices to remote clinics, in order to obtain injections of DMSO.

The Federal Drug Administration, and other governmental agencies in the United States, have been dead set against DMSO—blocking its sale as a prescriptive drug. Americans are now asking Congress to cancel these restrictions. Watch your newspapers!

While the fight over DMSO will soon be making headline news in print, it was actually television that fueled the fires and stirred up nationwide debate. "60 Minutes"—the top-rated news program on CBS-TV—did a special report on DMSO.

Mike Wallace interviewed Dr. Stanley Jacob, the leading spokesman for DMSO. The therapeutical effects of the drug were first discovered by Dr. Jacob in 1963. He and his associate—Robert Herschler, an organic chemist—did their research work in Oregon. Where the tall trees grow.

DMSO is derived from a substance which is found inside trees. It is called lignin, the material Nature uses to cement cells together within each tree.

You can apply DMSO topically—which means you just rub it on your skin. Dr. Jacob has proved that DMSO can penetrate the skin, travel through the bloodstream, and cause relief from pain. It works for many patients, people who suffer from a wide variety of injuries and ailments.

MY RESEARCH ON DMSO . . .

I wanted to make sure of the facts, before I recommended DMSO to any arthritics. First, I contacted the CBS television network. They provided me with a transcript of the "60 Minutes" broadcast. I have studied the script, and Mike Wallace lived up to his reputation. He fired difficult questions at Dr. Jacob . . . and he also talked with critics who were highly skeptical about DMSO.

Dr. Jacob passed this test with flying colors. Millions of TV viewers who watched that program are now firmly convinced that DMSO has real merit.

I know how Dr. Jacob felt that night. He was on the spot, facing Mike Wallace. I experienced the same type of interview years ago, early in my career as a nutrition theorist. At the time, the program was called "Nightbeat" . . . and Mike Wallace asked Dale Alexander some sharp, revealing questions. It's a form of cross-examination, an event you never forget.

Before writing these pages about DMSO, I decided to contact Dr. Jacob directly. To discuss with him, personally, the current status of his research on the drug. I found Dr. Jacob at the Oregon Health Sciences University in Portland. Here's what he told me . . .

The battle to achieve medical acceptance for DMSO *is* being won. Millions of people can now obtain it, legally, as a prescriptive drug—except in the United States.

In other countries, around the world, doctors and hospitals have been officially authorized to use this therapeutic substance.

Switzerland has approved DMSO as a prescriptive drug. For treating venous problems . . . and the Swiss also apply it topically (place it on the skin) as a *method to relieve bursitis and arthritis.*

Germany and Austria utilize DMSO, as a prescriptive drug, against acute and chronic musculoskeletal disorders.

Canada has accredited dimethyl sulfoxide for both topical and intravenous use against scleroderma.

Great Britain made DMSO prescriptive, together with IDU, for shingles.

I asked Dr. Jacob if there are any signs that DMSO will be certified in the United States. "Yes," he replied, "there are some favorable indications."

For example, the drug has already been approved for American doctors to use when their patients have interstitial cystitis. (Victims of this illness have a disabling inflammation of the urinary bladder.)

Dr. Jacob is also encouraged because DMSO has been granted further approval whereby it can be employed in the process of freezing blood platelets. These platelets can then be used during blood transfusions and other procedures in American hospitals.

DMSO, derived from wood pulp, was used for years merely as a solvent. A cleanser to remove paints and varnishes. Even today, the product can be manufactured inexpensively, for about four dollars a quart. But its medical use may have priceless benefits.

My main concern, of course, is to determine the value of DMSO in regard to arthritis. This drug may bring temporary relief. Evidence indicates that it is helpful in rejuvenating non-articular *membranes*. But I doubt whether it can help the *joint linings*. They still need lubricating oils. If your bodily joints are afflicted with rheumatoid arthritis, don't expect miracles from DMSO.

Dr. Jacob told me about an international conclave of doctors and scientists which will be held soon in Munich, Germany. He invited me to attend, so I can ask more questions about DMSO.

Yes, I shall make that trip to Germany. As part of my continuing investigation of DMSO. At this conference, I hope to find more answers about this drug. Then, I shall report the most pertinent facts, to arthritics everywhere.

STILL ANOTHER DISCOVERY . . . THE NEW VACCINE!

The momentous news came as a complete surprise. Even the way it was announced was most unusual. The first reports on this great medical discovery were released in those sensational tabloid newspapers which are found in supermarkets.

Millions of Americans, standing in line at check-out counters to pay for their groceries, saw the newspaper/magazines. Splashed on the cover of each publication were bold headlines:

"*MIRACLE VACCINE BEATS ARTHRITIS*" . . . you could read all about it in *The Globe*.

"*ARTHRITIS VACCINE . . . It could prevent and cure crippling disease.*" . . . said *The Star*.

According to the news stories, "*thanks to a major medical breakthrough just announced by top research scientists*" a revolutionary arthritis vaccine was now being developed that would end pain and suffering for millions of arthritics.

Like you, I quickly began reading these feature articles, filled with hope and optimism. If true, this was the biggest news of the century. Both of these dramatic stories quoted sources at the Scripps Clinic and Research Foundation in La Jolla, California. As an institution, there is none better in the world.

Located a few miles from San Diego, the Scripps Clinic is home base for several scientists—some very brilliant microbiologists and immunologists.

By reading the stories carefully, the public could understand some of the facts. The researchers have apparently discovered a way to regulate the immune system with antibodies produced in their laboratory.

The synthetic molecules (known as anti-idiotype antibodies) are able to force the immune system to destroy out-of-control antibodies—the kind that are believed to cause arthritis.

Dr. R.A. Houghten, at Scripps Clinic, reported

that eventually one method of controlling antibodies may be to administer an anti-arthritis injection. It would be similar to a "shot" given for tetanus after that disease strikes a person.

Another expert, quoted in the tabloid newspapers, was Dr. Richard Lerner. He discussed the work that he and his associates are doing at Scripps. Supposedly, according to the writer for the tabloid newspaper, Dr. Lerner said: "I feel very excited and confident this new method will rid people of rheumatoid arthritis."

MY SKEPTICAL REACTION . . .

The more I studied these news reports about the new "arthritis vaccine" it appeared that I should seek out *the real story*.

I promptly telephoned Dr. Houghton, at Scripps Clinic. He was not a happy man. He told me that the previous stories gave the wrong impression to the general public.

Vaccinations, to eliminate arthritis, are *not* "just around the corner" . . . the first steps have been taken, successfully, but it may take several *years* to develop this technique.

When I tried to reach Dr. Lerner by phone, he was refusing to speak with any more writers or reporters. He was so upset with journalists, that he won't talk anymore.

Apparently, the first stories were too optimistic, too soon. To say the least, the "announcement" of the miraculous vaccine was premature.

I will do some more investigative reporting . . . and I assure you I will stay on top of this story.

Finally, this week, through other contacts, I have been able to arrange an appointment for me to visit the Scripps Clinic. When I travel to La Jolla, I shall offer the doctors an opportunity to give me a more detailed account of exactly where they stand.

How much progress have they really made on creating and testing the arthritis vaccine?

Whatever they tell me, I shall pass on to you. Honestly and without exaggeration.

I'm still hopeful that Dr. Houghten and Dr. Lerner, or other men like them, can someday develop a "miracle drug" to eliminate arthritis. They are dedicated scientists who deserve our support and encouragement.

But there's still a long road ahead, and the discovery of that wonder drug may not happen in our lifetime.

That's why I shall continue my crusade to find a better answer, through nutrition.

I have been called an "Apostle of Good Health"—and I do speak fervently, like a man with a cause. During my lectures, I am apt to become enthusiastic. Some people say that I often sound like a preaching evangelist. If that be the case, let me quote the Bible.

These words (from Isaiah 1v 2) are the truth:

"Hearken diligently unto me and eat ye that which is good."

Like a missionary with a message, I shall continue to preach the doctrine of good nutrition . . . for the rest of my days.

CHAPTER VI

The Right Foods To Enjoy . . . Take Your Choice

Would you like some good news, for a change?

That last Chapter—about drugs that offer false hopes—was a little depressing. I suggest we talk about happier subjects. If you like delicious meals and tasty treats, these next few pages will offer you some pleasant surprises.

The diet I propose is permissive, easy to follow. You'll have a wide choice of foods—not a long list of restricted items.

You can still eat many of your favorite dishes. To help you recover from arthritis—through nutrition—the "cure" should not be worse than the disease. I shall not limit you to a strict diet. You won't have to follow some calorie-counting plan that borders on starvation.

I will ask, however, that you make a few changes in your eating habits. I'll name certain "oil-bearing" foods that you should try. Which meats and vegetables are best? I'll make specific suggestions . . . so you'll know what to look for at your local supermarket.

To cause arthritis pain to subside takes more than just cod liver oil. Your daily diet must also contribute nutritious elements. Take the first step, toward better health, by studying the next page . . .

THE "YES" LIST . . . FOODS ALLOWED AND RECOMMENDED

Arthritics who follow my dietary plan can choose any of the following foods. Select the best. . . .

FRUITS

Apples	Cantaloupe	Figs	Plums
Bananas	Casaba melon	Honeydew melon	Prunes
Blackberries	Cherries	Peaches	Raisins
Blueberries	Crenshaw melon	Pears	Raspberries
			Strawberries

(Fresh fruit, preferably. If in cans, drain off and discard the syrup. Sugar in juices is detrimental, if you have arthritis.)

VEGETABLES

Asparagus	Cauliflower	Escarole	Potatoes
Beans	Celery	Lettuce	Radishes
Beets	Chard	Lima beans	Spinach
Broccoli	Corn	Okra	Squash
Brussels sprouts	Cucumber	Onions	String beans
Cabbage	Eggplant	Peas	Tomatoes
Carrots	Endive	Peppers	Zucchini

FISH

Bluefish	Crab	Mackerel	Shrimp
Butterfish	Flounder	Oysters	Swordfish
Clams	Halibut	Pompano	Tuna
Cod	Lobster	Salmon	Trout
		Scallops	Whitefish

MEATS

Chicken	Lamb, leg of (lean)	Steak sirloin, porterhouse, top round, filet mignon, T-bone
Ham (lean)	Liver	Tongue
Hamburger (lean)	Pork (center cut, lean)	Turkey
Heart (beef)	Roast beef (lean)	Veal
Kidney		
Lamb chops (lean)		

DAIRY PRODUCTS

Cheese	Eggs
American	Milk
Blue cheese	(homogenized, Vitamin D., pasteurized, or raw certified), (Shake well.)
Cheddar	
Cottage	
Swiss	

For anyone with arthritis, the foods listed above are the most healthful. Use this page as a guide. You can enjoy everything from "A" to "Z" . . . from apples to zucchini. Cooking tips in Chapter XI.

You can see, immediately, that the list includes a wide variety of appetizing foods. I've placed very few limits on your choice of edibles. Because I am a firm believer in one doctrine: Eat well to be well!

As you begin my dietary program, in an effort to be helpful, I shall give you some suggested menus— for breakfast, lunch and dinner. (See Chapter XI).

Later, in this book, you'll even find a few of my favorite recipes. That's a bonus for the ladies—and for the male "gourmet cooks" who like to putter around in the kitchen.

But, seriously, I do want you to follow some basic rules concerning these foods. Don't overcook your meats and vegetables. Microwaving destroys many important enzymes . . . so I'll describe better methods of food preparation.

Think twice about what you eat and drink.

Realize, for example, that water is a food. It supplies your body with necessary minerals. But learn *when* to drink water . . . as I explain in the Menu Chapter.

Candy is a food. Eat it sparingly, but it's a source of carbohydrates. Giving you energy.

Cod liver oil is a food. It is rich in iodine. More important, it contains oil-soluble vitamins.

There I go again . . . praising the effectiveness of cod liver oil. Perhaps you would be convinced and share my enthusiasm for this oil if I show you what "osmosis" can do for arthritic joints.

We have already studied "digestion" and the

way oils are absorbed. (pages 30 to 36.) Now, let's see what actually happens *inside a joint cavity.*

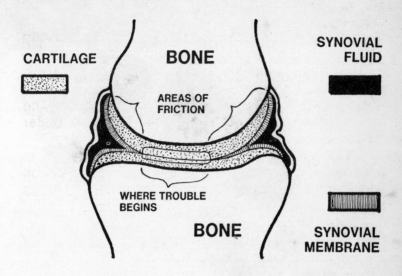

CARTILAGE

BONE

AREAS OF FRICTION

SYNOVIAL FLUID

WHERE TROUBLE BEGINS

BONE

SYNOVIAL MEMBRANE

WHERE "OSMOSIS" OCCURS WITHIN YOUR BODY

To better understand my theories on osmosis, just study this illustration. Locate the fluid in the joint (shown in solid black). Right next to it is a very thin area (marked with narrow vertical lines) to show the tissue lining known as the synovial membrane.

I maintain that cod liver oil, when it reaches this joint lining, is *metabolized* by the tissue lining.

The cod liver oil, as cod liver oil, does *not* get

into the joint fluid, within the joint cavity. Instead, the joint lining *takes from* the cod liver oil oil soluble Vitamin D and of helpful fatty acids——and converts them into mucin and hyaluronic acid.

When the cod liver oil is metabolized——creating mucin and hyaluronic acid——these two by-products begin to improve the viscosity of the joint fluid.

Throughout this book, I often refer to *viscosity*——which is the state of the fluid in any joint cavity. If it is viscous, the fluid is more sticky, adhesive and rope-like.

It generally takes three to six months of daily cod liver oil intake to upgrade the quality of the joint fluid viscosity.

Only then is the joint fluid capable of crossing the semi-permeable membrane ... and this process is known as *diffusion*. These substances (mucin and hyaluronic acid) which are diffused become valuable nutrition for the cartilage.

I am describing the only way that the cartilage can survive in a healthy form. *Absence of this kind of oil-augmented nutrition causes the cartilage to shrink. The thinner the cartilage becomes, the more osteoarthritis pain is experienced.* Why? Because much of the viscosity has left the joint fluid ... and the amount of fluid has diminished. So, the bones begin to rub against each other. This friction causes the pain.

THE PRIMARY REASON FOR OSTEOARTHRITIS

I define the problem of osteoarthritis very simply. The joint fluid is losing its viscosity——causing a narrowing of the joint space. The cartilage is also becoming thinner, unable to *cushion* bones.

> Your body can perform miraculous feats. This process of "osmosis" is one of them. Combine the facts on this page with what you have learned about digestion. REVIEW THE DRAWING ON PAGE 31

The pages you have just read——about the process of "osmosis"——contain indisputable facts. You must believe that osmosis will happen in the manner which I described. Otherwise, it makes no sense for you to follow my dietary program.

With these facts as a foundation, I proceeded to build my entire nutritional plan. Yes, the pages on osmosis are the "heart" of this book.

Success stories, from people who have tried my dietary approach, are most inspiring. I receive mail from arthritics of all ages. Women, men, and even children have gained healthful results.

Parents sometimes write to me. When I learn of any child, crippled with arthritis, I am saddened and

angered by the tragedy. For these families, perhaps I
can offer a few words of encouragement . . .

SUCCESS AGAINST JUVENILE RHEUMATOID ARTHRITIS

I am happy to report that some progress has
been made to alleviate arthritis when it strikes children. While writing this book, I consulted with many
medical authorities—including a famous pediatrician.

The expert on children's diseases whom I respect most is Lendon N. Smith, M.D., of Portland, Oregon. Among his accomplishments, he served for 25
years at Good Samaritan and Emanuel Hospitals in
Portland.

You may have seen Dr. Smith on television. The
TV networks hold him in high esteem—for the advice
he gives on matters of health. One indication of his
stature is the fact that he has been a guest on "The
Johnny Carson Show" a total of 42 times!

Recently, Dr. Smith and I were both invited to
give lectures at the annual convention of the National
Health Foundation. Following one lecture session, he
and I met privately. The two of us wanted to confer,
quietly. I sought answers . . . details about his method
of treating juvenile rheumatoid arthritis.

Dr. Smith told me about his years of pediatric
practice, back in Oregon. He diagnosed several
cases of this illness among young people, and he

would then refer these patients to a rheumatologist. As Dr. Smith tells it, that rheumatologist "used the standard aspirin, anti-inflammatories and often a course of a cortisone drug."

"All there was to offer," says Dr. Smith, "was medicine to relieve pain and physiotherapy to discourage stiffness. After I moved to a nutritional approach to diseases, I was called by parents who wanted a more comprehensive intervention rather than just symptom relief."

Dr. Smith tried to help the juveniles through a nutritional program. He augmented their diet by providing them with additional amounts of Vitamin C, calcium, magnesium, B complex vitamins, etc. He supplied his patients with Vitamin D (500 to 1,000 units) and Vitamin A (5,000 to 10,000 units) *usually as cod liver oil.*

"I made them stop the sugar, the white flour . . ." Dr. Smith reports. "I was shoring up their adrenal glands, so the patients could get well more naturally."

(Does this plan of action sound familiar? Yes, it is very close to the approach which I have been recommending for 35 years!)

In conclusion, Dr. Smith made this statement: "The results came slowly, but the attacks of fever and swollen joints appeared less frequently and were less severe."

What wonderful words those are! *"Swollen joints appeared less frequently and were less severe."*

Someday, soon, that kind of improvement can be yours. If you correct your diet and select the foods shown on page 57.

To be sure, you should also observe a few rules regarding the beverages you drink. Don't "dilute" the benefits you gain from good foods by gulping down too many liquids.

Some beverages you can consume, in moderation . . . others you should avoid.

Think, then drink. My common sense advice on this topic begins on the next page . . .

CHAPTER VII

Coffee, Tea, Soda Pop . . . What About Allergies?

Millions of Americans are gulping down coffee, cup after cup, almost like addicts.

Millions of families, throughout the British Isles, are quaffing too much tea.

Millions of children, worldwide, are guzzling soda pop at a rate that's insane.

I would be guilty of a glaring omission if I failed to include in this book some urgent warnings about these beverages. So, in this chapter, I shall offer my special comments about these popular drinks.

Actually, I am not going to tell you to *stop* drinking coffee and tea. On the contrary, I am merely going to suggest some common sense rules on *how* and *when* to enjoy "a cuppa coffee" or "a spot of tea." I'll even report on some alternative liquids. They taste like your favorite brew . . . yet they are healthy additions to your diet.

Let's examine the leading thirst-quenchers, one at a time . . .

COFFEE . . . PLAIN AND DECAFFEINATED

You may continue to drink coffee, even if you have arthritis, as long as you consume it ten minutes *before* a meal. If taken with this "time cushion" for your digestive system, then damage is minimal.

By separating your coffee intake from the meal itself, then the caffeine and other elements in coffee will not cause any drying effect in your body.

I do not see any particular advantage in drinking decaffeinated coffee. Unfortunately, the process used to decaffeinate the coffee beans requires the addition of new chemicals—which often cause added toxicity and can adversely affect your liver and kidneys.

For the least harm to your system, if you are an arthritic, I suggest that you drink your coffee black. Heavy use of cream and sugar complicates rheumatoid arthritis specifically, because it causes more rapid deterioration of an already sensitive joint lining.

Another word of caution: If you use a non-dairy product in your coffee, you should realize that this substance is usually about 65% sugar. Avoid all such substitutes.

Perhaps a better plan for coffee-lovers is to try making a switch to a health food product. There are coffee-like substitutes now on the market which are composed primarily of malt and barley. Instead of being made from coffee beans, these are powdered extracts. Several blends are manufactured in Germany, where the grains are grown especially for this purpose.

TEA TIME . . . A HABIT THAT'S SPREADING

We all smile about one British tradition. You've heard how, at a certain time each day, Englishmen all stop work to enjoy a cup of tea. (The fact is, they stop several times daily, for tea. Which is no different than Americans, who take a lot of "coffee breaks.")

I'm all for this idea . . . I have savored "tea and crumpets" during all my trips to Great Britain. The popularity of tea is growing, throughout the world, so let me make a few simple suggestions. Some guidelines for arthritics . . .

You can drink tea, but please do it at the right time. Ideally, that's ten minutes before any meal—or at least four hours after a meal. Remember that tea is a liquid with "high surface tension" and it should not be allowed to conflict with the digestion of oil-bearing foods.

The potential problem with tea is most severe in the British Isles. Because much of the tea consumed in England is grown in India—and this type, which they import, has a very high concentration of tannic acid.

Tannic acid has a drying effect on the linings of our bodily joints. So, arthritics, be forewarned.

Dry skin is evident among tea-drinkers, resulting in "crow's feet" near the eyes. I maintain that too much tannic acid is responsible. Britishers also brew this beverage with an abundance of loose tea leaves, for stronger taste. That's another complicating factor.

Across the world, in Japan, again we find millions of people drinking tea. But the Japanese prefer a much milder type. They use smaller amounts, served in tiny cups. And, usually, they drink it without sugar.

In the United States, the addiction to tea has started to mushroom. While most Americans use the milder forms of tea, we go overboard in adding sugar. Then, in summer months, we commit a worse sin by dropping ice cubes into the tea! Iced beverages are suicidal.

The cubes, in a glass of iced tea, will definitely hinder the assimilation process. They fight with your dietary oils.

Herbal tea is a better alternative.

Many readers of my previous books have already discovered the advantages of herbal tea. The pleasing taste has converted millions of people to this drink. It has the natural healing power of herbs, with no additives and no preservatives.

You have your choice of flavors—like cinnamon, peppermint, rose hips, orange blossom, etc.

Instead of sugar, try adding some honey. For sweetening, I've sometimes used a teaspoon of apple or cherry concentrate. Herbal tea has always been available in health food stores. Today, it has become so popular that many supermarkets now stock this product.

A HORROR STORY . . . WE'RE DROWNING IN SODA POP!

To help you win your war against arthritis I may have to frighten you. Scare you into taking action, so you will pay more attention to your daily diet. That's why I'm now going to write a grim and shocking report about carbonated beverages.

You face an enormous threat to your health, if you are hooked on "soft" drinks. Yes, we are becoming addicts, unable to resist the fizzy liquids. This habit is taking a terrible toll, causing health problems among adults and children.

Too many people think that the soda pop craze is limited to youngsters. Not so. Even senior citizens are now quenching their thirst by reaching for a can of cola—or some other bubbly concoction.

For the older folks, it all seems innocent enough. They are not drinking liquor. They're just enjoying "soft" drinks.

Well, let me say, most emphatically, there is nothing "soft" about soda pop. Those bottles and six-packs contain harsh, harmful ingredients. Arthritics, in particular, are courting disaster if they don't avoid carbonated liquids.

The extent of this national problem is astonishing. Do you realize how much money Americans spent on soft drinks, in just one year? The total is $24,498,364,000. That's 24 *billion* dollars!

I contacted the United States Department of Agriculture to obtain these facts. The Economics and Research Division stated that the latest statistics available are for the year of 1982. And here's the horrifying proof of our addiction to soda pop. In that year, we consumed 6,686,181,000 packaged *gallons* of soft drinks.

More than six *billion* gallons ... what a sad commentary on the way we ignore our health, until pain attacks.

I am not alone, in my condemnation of carbonated beverages. Many distinguished doctors have publicly denounced these soft drinks. One comprehensive report, surveying several experts, was published in *Let's Live* Magazine. They blamed soda pop as a possible cause for sleeplessness, nightmares, behavioral disturbances, indigestion, burning urine, hyperactivity, cavities, and a wide variety of other ailments.

Among the physicians whom the magazine quoted was a highly-skilled allergist, Dr. Marshall Mandell. (To learn more about his background and his exceptional qualifications, see pages 74 to 76 of this book. He was discussing the potential hazards lurking in bottles and cans.

"Look at the contents," said Dr. Mandell. "You have artificial coloring, artificial flavoring, preservatives and sugar.

"First of all, you have simple bad nutrition and

drainage of health from all that sugar. It comes into the system as empty calories, bringing no nutrients with it. The soda pop actually has to steal from vitamins, minerals and enzymes already in the body in order to metabolize.

"Then you have the allergic reactions. People can be sensitive to any of the components, to the cane sugar, the corn sugar, the artificial coloring or artificial flavoring.

"We have tested perhaps 150 to 200 children and in many cases found something in soda pop as the cause of an allergic response.

"The coloring, for instance, is made from coal tar, and people who are chemically reactive to it can have all kinds of trouble.

"We've seen people react with arthritic pains, generalized itching, an attack of asthma, or a migraine. We've seen kids get confused, angry, and go into a bizarre hyperactive state, pushing furniture around, striking their parents and running up and down the hall screaming.

"We saw a case where a child could drink one brand of orange soda and nothing happened. But when he drank another brand, it contained a different ingredient that made him wild and uncontrollable."

Continuing his report on actual case histories, the allergist said: "We had another patient who was diagnosed with a 'nervous bladder.' She had to urinate 15 times a day. Her problem was cola beverages and chocolate, and when we got her off those, her condition completely cleared up."

I'll have more to say about allergies shortly. But,

first, no discussion about "drinking" would be complete until we cover the topics of liquor and beer.

Alcoholic beverages, for adults with arthritis, are permissible—providing you take certain precautions. You can enjoy an occasional highball or cocktail. Just be sure to drink it at least 10 minutes before eating—not during your meals.

Your goal is to keep that liquor away from your dietary oil while your foods are being digested.

Oddly enough, it is preferable that arthritics should take their drinks straight ... or with plain water. Do not "mix" with carbonated beverages. Even club soda has an acidity rating of 4.7 and causes your digestive system to work harder, slowing the assimilation of your foods.

Beer is bottled with carbonation to make it foam. That gives it bad marks in my book. For good health, please limit your beer drinking as much as possible. At the very least, wait until three hours after mealtime before imbibing.

I have stated my case. If you give up carbonated beverages, you can avoid allergies and many illnesses. Why trade your health for a few fizzy drinks!

ALLERGIES ... THEIR RELATION TO ARTHRITIS

When a person develops an allergy to one or several specific foods, this reaction is frequently a warning sign of impending arthritis. The allergic condition is usually characterized by symptoms in some or many parts of the body, including the joints and muscles.

Allergic people, especially those with rheumatoid and osteoarthritis, often have problems in their digestive and respiratory tracts as well as their nervous systems. Their symptoms include colitis with constipation, diarrhea and cramps; asthma with coughing, wheezing and shortness of breath; migraine headaches with nausea and vomiting; and fatigue.

Different combinations of these afflictions are commonly experienced by millions of arthritics because they suffer from bodywide allergy.

Prominent doctors, some of the leading allergists in America and worldwide, are starting to link allergies with arthritis and are attempting to treat both ailments simultaneously.

The present methods of detecting allergies in human beings have been greatly improved and are much more accurate; they have become an exact science. Back in the 1940's, when I began studying health subjects, allergists would "scratch" or inject test solutions into a patient's arm to cause mosquito bite like "wheals" on the skin. The accepted tests were to introduce certain food, dust, pollen or mold extracts into a person, and then look for "reactions".

For many people "having an allergy" means getting the sneezes and sniffles. Another common complaint is the occurrence of red, itching, watery eyes when certain pollens or dandruff (dander) from house pets is in the air. Perhaps you, or someone you

know, will experience an allergic affliction——like
breaking out with itchy hives. Or, you might develop
puffy eyelids and lips.

If you contract any such ailment, go to an allergist. Let him inspect the condition and diagnose the
cause.

Now, in the 1980's, there is a much more accurate symptom-duplicating allergy-testing technique. A
number of progressive allergists are using this new
method. It is known as sublingual (under-the-tongue)
provocative testing. Allergenic extracts are placed
under the tongue. They are very rapidly absorbed into
the circulation and reach all parts of the body.

The sites where allergic reactions occur will
flare up, and the patient's familiar symptoms will be
reproduced——showing exactly how the substance affects each person. This method of testing is far more
effective than skin or blood tests.

One noted allergist who has used this sublingual
procedure very succesfully is Marshall Mandell, M.D.,
the Medical Director of the New England Foundation
for Allergic and Environmental Diseases. (The Foundation is located in Norwalk, Connecticut.)

Dr. Mandell has employed the sublingual technique in more than 1,000,000 tests during the past
20 years!

A well-trained allergist can usually trace the
cause in complicated cases. When it's from eating to-
matoes, or eggs, or fish, or strawberries, many times
the cause is easily detected by the patient.

But I want to discuss a much more serious form
of internal allergy——*the allergic reactions to food and*

beverages that occur in and around joints. That painful affliction is now sometimes identified as "allergic-arthritis".

The damage caused when you contantly consume carbonated soft drinks is enormous. I also deplore the harm you do to yourself when you flood your digestive system with sugar, "caffeine" and tannic acid, by drinking too many glasses of iced tea.

By making nutritional errors like these, you decrease the overall quality of your health. You lower your resistance and become a candidate for allergies to develop.

Worse, by eating too many wrong foods—or too much of the "right" foods—the nutritional damage and allergic over-loading by such foods can pass your body's threshold of tolerance. The result can be allergies in different parts of the body, some of which can be *very* uncomfortable. An arthritic may experience a local or generalized *reaction* in and around the joints. Painful inflammation can develop in the surrounding muscle, and severe fatigue can also occur.

A NEW TERM: ALLERGIC-ARTHRITIS

Due to some important scientific pioneering, the term "allergic-arthritis" has now come into popular usage. This is a general description which is being applied to many common forms of arthritis.

Earlier in this chapter, I mentioned Dr. Mandell. He is the acknowledged expert on these diseases.

In addition to being a physician, Dr. Mandell is a

Diplomate of the American Board of Allergy and Immunology. His prestigious credentials also include being a Fellow of the American College of Allergists.

I found myself in agreement with Dr. Mandell on several points when I read about his allergy-based studies of "Bio-ecologic" disorders. He has often stated in his writings that *good nutrition* is essential in the fight against arthritis.

For laymen and the general public, he recently wrote a self-help book. The title is: "Dr. Mandell's Lifetime Arthritis Relief System" (published by Coward-McCann.) I strongly suggest that you read it.

Dr. Mandell urges removing the dietary allergens and eliminating or controlling the environmental substances that are causing or flaring up arthritis. And, then, he recommends *"supporting the patient internally by means of superior nutrition."*

Such a plan of action will also make the arthritic person less susceptible to illness in general.

I respect this eminent allergist. So, I truly appreciate the comments he made about me. Dr. Mandell wrote the Foreword to this book. (See pages 1–3.)

You have learned, in these past few pages, that allergies can be a serious problem for arthritics. If you do become afflicted, you'll have plenty of company. Many celebrities—who appear in Hollywood films and on TV—have been victims of allergic ailments.

One famous case is covered in the next chapter . . . the tale of "The Sports Star and His Chocolate Bars!"

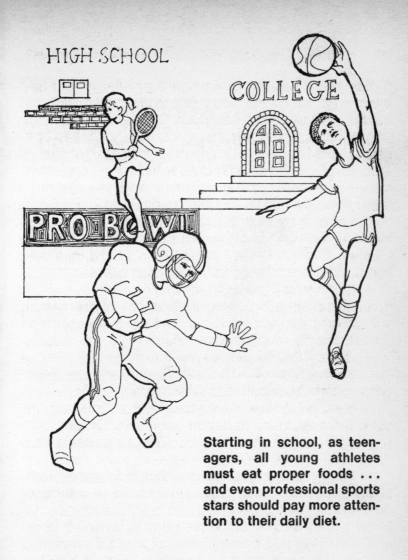

HIGH SCHOOL

COLLEGE

PRO BOWL

Starting in school, as teen-agers, all young athletes must eat proper foods ... and even professional sports stars should pay more attention to their daily diet.

In the next chapter, we examine the role of
NUTRITION IN SPORTS MEDICINE . . .

CHAPTER VIII

Sports Medicine . . . How You Can Benefit

As I sit at my typewriter, ready to write this chapter, my mind goes forth to a faraway village in the nation of Greece. The nightly newscasts on TV are featuring stories about the citizens of Olympia who are preparing to light that flaming torch which signals the start of the Olympics.

Soon, athletes from around the globe will be competing for Gold Medals . . . as we all applaud and share their spirit of national pride.

I am also fascinated by the mental picture of joggers and runners. Thousands of them have volunteered to help carry the Olympic torch, as they run in relays from Olympia, Greece, all the way to Los Angeles. (Later in this chapter I will have some comments about marathon runners. We can all learn from their experience, because many of them have suffered from aching muscles and damaged knee joints. They also know which foods to consume to gain maximum energy.)

It's no secret. I'm a sports fan. Baseball, football, hockey, you name it. As long as I can *sit* and watch.

In the course of my travels, as a nutrition theorist, I have made many friends in the world of

sports. I have known famous athletes and TV sports-
casters. I've also been interviewed by leading newspaper columnists whose bylines are featured on the
Sports Pages.

I am very grateful for the time they have spent
with me, and for the friendly interest they have shown
in my dietary theories. To indicate just some of my activities in the field of athletics, let me quote two newspaper articles by well-known sportswriters. Here are
some excerpts, from clippings I saved in my scrapbook.

First, there's a humorous column, written by Jim
Murray of *The Los Angeles Times*. Very appropri-
ately, the headline reads *Some Food For Thought.*
The story concerns the New York Yankees. Yogi
Berra was having problems, possibly caused by poor
diet. So, his coach, Casey Stengel, came to the res-
cue . . .

Quoting from a column in *The Los Angeles Times* . . .

Casey called in nutritionist Dan Dale Alexander,
a man whose surest diagnostic tool is the handshake.
Most doctors peer down the throat or check the eyes.
Dale Alexander checks the grip. If the hand is cold,
the rest of you soon will be.

Yogi's hands were not only cold, they were
scaly. It was like shaking hands with a fish. Yogi had
eczema. "He couldn't grip a bat, his anxious hands
itched so."

Dale Alexander soon saw the trouble. Scattered

around the room were empty bottles of chocolate milk. Yogi drank it by the case. The more he drank, the drier his skin became. Pretty soon, not even golf gloves could help at the bat. Yogi was batting .220, and was itchier than a hound dog.

Alexander says he took Yogi off the chocolate and onto cod-liver oil. Dale Alexander thinks cod-liver oil can cure anything from the common cold to falling hair, from arthritis, to arteriosclerosis and, probably, the Johnstown flood. In any case, it cured Yogi's batting average. He ended up the season at .296 and not a scratch on him.

————————

Another columnist, very popular in the Chicago area, is Jack Mabley. He told his readers the true story of my work with Ernie Banks, when he was with the Chicago Cubs baseball team. They were playing the Dodgers, in Los Angeles, when this incident occurred . . .

Quoting from a column in *The Chicago Tribune* . . .

Dale Alexander, a nutritionist, walked into the Los Angeles Dodgers' clubhouse to see Ernie Banks and shuddered. "A nutritional disaster," Alexander exclaimed. "Chocolate bars everywhere. Athletes should never be permitted near chocolate bars."

Banks' friend Billy Williams had suggested that Ernie see Alexander about his bum knees. Alexander said Ernie drank too much tea—vats of it, hot or iced. "Tannin in tea is used to cure leather," Alexander said. "That gives you an idea of how powerful its action is on tissue."

After he got Banks to switch to cod liver oil from tea, Alexander said, his knees were as good as new in 60 days . . ."

(When I met columnist Jack Mabley, it was in his office at *The Chicago Tribune.* I was already past 60 years of age, but I was in robust good health, and I was brimming over with enthusiasm.)

. . . Alexander comes on as a bit eccentric, and he has no degree letters after his name. His main credentials are five books on health, one of which, "Arthritis and Common Sense," led the national best sellers for several weeks.

. . . "I've got the skin of a baby," he beamed as he rubbed his cheeks with both hands. "And this hair," he added, pointing to a monk's ring around his shining dome, "is all new. I didn't have a hair on my head for 40 years."

(I then told the Jack Mabley my main message. While praising the value of cod liver oil, I also admitted that I can't even stand the smell of the stuff.)

. . . Alexander says it got a bad reputation because it was taken straight, by the spoonful. Now you can get it in cherry flavor or as part of a milk shake or in all kinds of other disguises.

His theory is that the body needs lubricating oil, just as an engine does. He says the oil must get into the bloodstream instead of going first though the liver.

The key to sending the natural oil in our foods to

the bloodstream is to escort them with oil-bearing liquids during and after eating, he says. Whole milk and soup qualify.

Not qualifying, he says, are skim milk, coffee, tea, soft drinks, liquor, wine, and ice cubes.

I can't see any mad rush for milk and soup by lovers of coffee, tea, soft drinks, and booze. But Alexander swears this is the way to better health.

————————

Like many people, I bet on the outcome of sports events. I gamble. In fact, this past year I wagered a grand total of five dollars. A friend of mine wanted to bet me $5.00 on a football game. It was the Super Bowl, and he let me choose my favorite team. Okay, I'll admit it. I lost the $5.00—"but wait'll next year!"

Speaking of football, let me tell a brief story about a gridiron superstar. Roman Gabriel was making Sports Page headlines—as quarterback of the Philadelphia Eagles—when this incident began.

Gabriel was having painful problems affecting one of his knees. As he traveled with the team, he read two of my books—including an earlier edition of "Arthritis and Common Sense." The football star wrote to me personally, and mailed the letter to my Publisher. It was forwarded to me, because I was on a lecture tour in Canada.

I telephoned Roman Gabriel, and we talked. It happened that I was scheduled to lecture in Philadelphia about three weeks later. We arranged to meet.

When I arrived in the City of Brotherly Love, I went out to the football field where the team was practicing. Roman Gabriel asked me many questions about foods, menus, and cod liver oil. He decided to try my dietary program. About three months later he was pain-free—and able to continue his stellar football career!

We are friends to this day. I talked with Roman Gabriel, in Phoenix, Arizona, this month. He is now an outstanding quarterback coach, working for George Allen and the *Arizona Wranglers,* in the new United States Football League.

These last few pages—about professional baseball and football players—could teach the team owners an important lesson.

The giant athletic organizations sign players to multi-million dollar contracts. To protect their roster of stars, the teams have resident physicians, resident surgeons, trainers, therapists, even astrologers and psychiatrists—*but never nutritionists!*

I am baffled as to why proper diet is not considered as a prime requirement to keep athletes healthy.

A vast series of ailments—ranging from tendinitis to ham-string muscles to rheumatic pain—could be avoided. Team managers must pay more attention to what their players *eat* and *drink.* Drying up of the joints will run more people out of a football league than hard tackles by Lyle Alzado!

ONE DOCTOR WHO UNDERSTANDS . . . A PATHOLOGIST

I was encouraged to read, not long ago, some comments by Thomas J. Bassler, M.D., which indicated his awareness of foods and diet as a means to accomplish better health.

Dr. Bassler is now doing important work in the Department of Pathology at Centinela Hospital in Inglewood, California. He is nationally known for his research among marathon runners—one of the sports which is always highlighted during the Olympics. Dr. Bassler is currently conducting a study involving 159 marathoners. Some of them ran 10 kilometers (6 miles) and others raced 42 kilometers regularly—more than 26 miles!

Naturally, many of the long distance runners contract muscular and skeletal damage . . . sometimes to the point where they require "orthotic" devices to help treat injuries to their heels, feet or knees.

(Here is a simple definition of "orthotics" . . . It is the science of developing and fitting surgical devices to activate or supplement a weakened limb. In other words, the use of splints, elastic bandages, braces, etc.)

I decided to meet with Dr. Bassler, because of something he wrote. It was an excellent article which was published in *Sports Medicine* magazine. He stated, in print: "Runners with rheumatoid symptoms may benefit from orthotics, however *their nutritional needs should not be overlooked.*"

Writing for podiatrists—whose patients are faced with articular tissue problems—Dr. Bassler reported on the value of linoleic acid. I agree that this fatty acid (linoleic) is essential for better health. I recommend certain foods as good sources of linoleic acid. That's one reason why you should include fish, beans, whole grains and other vegetables in your diet.

I traveled to Dr. Bassler's hospital to confer with him personally. We discussed the fact that arachidonic acid is one of three fatty acids that are found in cod liver oil. I indicated to him that this fatty acid in this oil could be superior to linoleic . . . even more beneficial for marathon runners, to give them freer joint movement.

We discussed what causes long-distance runners to "tire out." What are the right foods to make them "last" longer, with a "kick" at the finish line?

Dr. Bassler told me, in his opinion, red meats were the best energizers. However, he has found that vegetarians often have more "zip" in the early stages of a marathon race.

This is the same Dr. Bassler who has done notable research on the causes of heart disease. He has recent evidence that poor nutrition is a contributing factor in atherosclerosis. Briefly, let me summarize some of his views on ASCVD—the illness known to millions of people as "hardening of the arteries."

MISTAKES WHICH LEAD TO ATHEROSCLEROSIS

A too rich diet, lack of exercise, and tobacco use . . . these are three key errors which Dr. Bassler warns against. If you want to ward off hardening of the arteries, read these next few paragraphs carefully.

Dr. Bassler prepared a medical paper, and it was published in the *Annals of the New York Academy of Sciences.* He made this statement: "The urban diet is suspect because it lacks food "fiber," unsaturated fats, ascorbic acid, and tocopherols."

("Tocopherol" is an alcohol having the properties of Vitamin E. It is isolated from wheat germ oil, or can be produced synthetically.)

The medical report went on to discuss the healthy physical condition of the Masai warriors who live in Africa. They travel great distances, herding cattle on foot, and they seldom suffer from the heart diseases which are common among "civilized" people. The primitive tribesmen eat a natural diet. They are lucky . . . they have *no* refined foods.

Autopsies have been performed on these African warriors. Pathologists found that the coronary arteries of the Masai were enlarged, making them less susceptible to atherosclerosis.

Other scientists have conducted tests based on the diet of the Tarahumara ("Flying Feet") Indians of northern Mexico. Since the days of Montezuma and the Aztec empire, they have been known for their marathon running. They jog through the jungles, in the heat of high noon.

In their village, these Indians stage ceremonial "runs"—and their physical fitness has been attributed to their antiatherogenic diet. They live in a fertile valley. In the productive soil, they grow corn and beans. Natural foods. (One nutritional study included 372 Tarahumara Indians, a sizeable sampling of their dietary habits.)

SOME "HEARTENING" FACTS ABOUT ESKIMOS

The sport of dog-sledding is a grueling test of man's strength and stamina. As they race across the Arctic snow, each sled driver faces bitter cold winds . . . and I marvel at their endurance as I watch them on TV.

I admire the Eskimo people, for another reason. They are among the most healthy individuals in the world. For generations, they have *not* suffered from arthritis. And, to them, atherosclerosis is extremely rare.

I think I know why . . .

Eskimos have always eaten an abundance of fish. *Marine fish oils* have helped keep them warm and strong.

Their robust good health has been legendary. But, then, some Eskimos began to migrate to Canada to enjoy the "benefits" of civilization. When they adopted a diet containing refined foods and carbonated soft drinks, they started to suffer from cardiovascular disease and arthritis.

As long as the Eskimos were eating their normal meals, they never had to worry about hardening of the arteries. Because there is a substance in marine fish oil known as EPA.

(This abbreviation, EPA, stands for eicosapentanoic acid.) Some scientists report that this fatty acid can help lower cholesterol and triglyceride levels in the blood. I repeat, *cod liver oil contains generous amounts of EPA.*

During a research study done at the Oregon Health Sciences Center, a doctor placed patients on a fish diet. It produced beneficial chemical changes in their bloodstreams, including drops in cholesterol.

I have read several reports which substantiate these facts. A different group of patients followed their doctor's advice. He changed them from polyunsaturated vegetable oils to cod liver oil. Result: "The tendency of their platelets to aggregate and adhere to blood vessel walls appears to have been reduced——making it more difficult for blood clots to form."

Some physicians still question the merits of cod liver oil. They act surprised when I extoll the many advantages of this oil. They accuse me of proposing some "new-fangled plan" to reduce cholesterol.

Don't they realize that serious research began 25 years ago!

Way back in 1959, in October, the United States Department of the Interior reported the results of some extensive studies which they authorized. Across the nation, it was headline news: *"RE-SEARCH PROVES VALUE OF FISH BODY OIL IN REDUCING CHOLESTEROL LEVELS."*

The scientific investigations were conducted by the Bureau of Commercial Fisheries, Fish and Wildlife Service, with the cooperation of the Hormel Institute of the University of Minnesota. The news story said:

"A 'saturated' fat, such as lard, congreals at low temperatures. An 'unsaturated' fat does not congeal readily. This is the property which permits oil-laden fish to move freely in waters of low temperature.

"Bureau research has shown that about half of the body oil of most species of fish is unsaturated and about 10 per cent of it is highly unsaturated. This latter portion of the fish oil contains five or six unsaturated carbon atoms per 'chain,' compared with only two such atoms in vegetable oil. In other words the potential of fish oil in reducing the cholesterol level is approximately three times that of vegetable oils."

Millions of people saw and read that news story. I wish a few more doctors had.

Enough said. I have given you my heartfelt advice on atherosclerosis. Now, let's return to the topic of athletes . . . and the wide, wide world of sports.

RACQUETBALL IS THE LATEST FAD

Everywhere you look, these days, new clubhouses are being built. They feature classes on physical fitness—and cement courts for playing racquetball.

Hundreds of thousands of Americans, young and old, are paddling racquetballs at breakneck speed. The sport is now the "in" thing, the right lifestyle.

There is an inspiring sidelight to the racquetball craze. Perhaps you have read about it . . . the true story of a girl named Lynn Adams.

A popular magazine published the facts, told how 26-year-old Lynn has been a victim of rheumatoid arthritis for many years. But she has triumphed over the disease. She loved to play racquetball, and she kept practicing this sport even though her hands, knees and other bodily joints were often hit by painful attacks of arthritis.

Finally, despite her agony, Lynn Adams began to compete on the women's professional racquetball circuit. She now earns $75,000 a year as a sports star. She has even attained the top title. Lynn is the Women's World Racquetball Champion!

There is hope for arthritics . . . and Lynn Adams is proving it!

DOCTORS NOW "SPECIALIZE" IN SPORTS MEDICINE

There are more than *one million* sports injuries in the United States each year, 100,000 of them involving children.

To meet this epidemic of accidents, the medical profession has started to train doctors who will be especially skilled to serve these casualties. An official name has been adopted: SPORTS MEDICINE . . . the science of preventing, treating and rehabilitating sports injuries. So far, so good.

But I want to make a vital suggestion. This time, will organized medicine please make sure that all these new doctors are also taught some basic facts about *nutrition.*

Proper foods and menus can have a reparative value, as an athlete recovers from torn ligaments. There are ways to combat Achilles' heel or "tennis elbow" through natural nutrition.

Already the field of sports medicine includes orthopedic surgeons, podiatrists, chiropractors, dentists and psychologists. All I ask is that these learned experts also inquire about the eating habits of each patient.

Some progress is being made, as this chapter has demonstrated. Scientists study the Eskimos, and explore the diets of Indian marathon runners in Mexico. But it is time to expand these efforts. In our search for nutritional knowledge, let's use the facilities of colleges and medical schools, worldwide.

In the title of this Chapter, I spoke of "How You Can Benefit" from sports medicine. The fact is you are already reaping the rewards. Every time a doctor examines the aching joints of an athlete, he is trying to solve problems that are closely related to arthritis. Discoveries *have* been made, and more will come . . . to aid arthritics.

Meanwhile, let's all follow the careers of our favorite athletes, for sheer enjoyment. Root for the high school basketball team, cheer for a college football hero. Play golf. For many of us, sports can be the best medicine.

KEEP YOUR pH <u>UP</u>

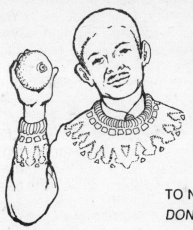

The NORMAL pH of the saliva in your mouth should be 7.0 to 7.1

CHEW ACID FRUITS

TO NEUTRALIZE THEM

DON'T BY-PASS YOUR SALIVA

ALKALINE

7

6

5

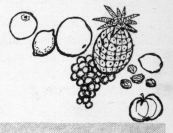

4

3 If the above fruits are not

2 chewed, then they will fall below the 4.5 acidity level

1

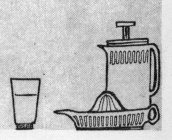

ACID

93

CHAPTER IX

Avoid Acidity . . . And Use Vitamins Wisely

At each of my lectures—when I invite questions from the audience—there are two topics which seem to puzzle many arthritics.

First, they all want to know my attitude toward citrus fruit. Most everyone admits that they drink fruit juices frequently. Is that a good idea?

Second, when victims of arthritis are speaking freely, they often raise questions about the value of taking vitamin pills. I am always asked for my honest opinion regarding vitamin supplements.

No wonder so many people are somewhat confused by these matters. For years the citrus industry has promoted their juices as a great source of Vitamin C. Meanwhile, pharmaceutical companies are constantly introducing newly concocted multi-vitamin capsules.

Perhaps, in this chapter, I can address both of these issues. I shall dispel some myths, separate fact from fiction. I shall now report on why you face *potential problems* due to citric acids . . . and how you can gain *potential advantages* from certain vitamins.

If you have arthritis, don't ignore the dangers of acidity. Take some preventive measures, as shown in the drawing on page 93. I urge you to "keep your pH up!" Let me explain that statement . . .

Chemists and scientists use the letters "pH" as a symbol to help designate the degree of acidity in a liquid.

They have established that water has a pH of 7. (Approximately 10,000,000 quarts of water contain one gram of hydrogen ion "acid"—and, in mathematics, the logarithm of 10,000,000 is seven.) So, when measuring acids in foods or liquids, anything which registers above 7 is alkaline, and below 7 is acid.

From that mid-point of 7, the scale which denotes acidity descends *downward. The lower the pH, the more acid in that food or beverage.*

Lemon juice has the worst rating, in terms of acidity. Scientific tests—to determine the acid content and how caustic it is—proved that lemon juice has a very negative pH of 2.29.

Grapefruit juice is nearly as bad, because it registers a pH level of 2.98.

Orange juice is 3.42 and tomato juice has a pH of 4.18.

If you drink "high-acid" liquids—too profusely and too often—you will soon have a "gassy stomach" and other discomforts. More serious symptoms can also develop, like nausea and ulcers.

When you eat or drink too many acidic foods, you force your blood and your digestive system to work extra hard *to neutralize those acids.* For instance, your body "borrows" mineral salts from your blood and tissues to counteract the increased acidity.

"Rob" your tissues in this manner, and they can start to degenerate. Result: a prelude to arthritis.

For all these reasons, you should learn your personal "acidity rating" . . . so you can *maintain* your pH at a normal level.

A simple measuring device, to determine pH, is now available at most drugstores. It is an inexpensive "kit" containing small strips of nitrazine paper. You place a tiny strip, about the size of a matchstick, under your tongue. In just 10 or 15 seconds, the paper changes color—it records the degree of acidity in your saliva. As a rule, any healthy person will register from 6.0 to 7.

CHEW MORE! YOUR SALIVA CAN COMBAT THOSE ACIDS!

When you swallow highly acidic foods, without chewing them thoroughly, you have cheated yourself. You have by-passed your saliva . . . preventing it from serving its true purpose.

Nature gave us saliva, as a key element in our digestive system. It can soften and "dilute" our foods, and help dissipate the acidity in whatever we eat. If you gulp down your foods, it is an unhealthy habit. *Don't ignore the chewing and salivating process.*

In fact, I even recommend citrus fruits as part of

your diet. As long as you *chew* the fruit. Peel a fresh orange, and enjoy eating it! But stop guzzling glassfuls of citric juices. Don't flood your stomach with ice-cold acidic beverages.

In these past two pages I have spoken harshly about citrus products. I condemn their acid content. I have always said, however, that you can consume *limited amounts* of orange juice in a beneficial way.

Mixing orange juice with cod liver oil creates a perfect blend of healthful products. This method, combining both substances, I have recommended for more than 30 years!

The orange juice is "emulsified" with the oil, and both become easily absorbed.

I have never questioned the fact that orange juice is rich in Vitamin C. That's a great advantage, not to be missed.

The time has come, in this book manuscript, for a frank discussion about several different vitamins. Here are my very specific comments . . .

THE TRUTH ABOUT VITAMINS . . . FOR VICTIMS OF ARTHRITIS

In medical circles, among many doctors, a debate continues. Some physicians are not ready to prescribe vitamins for their arthritic patients. Vitamin D is sometimes credited with having a supporting role

. . . but arthritis, as a disease, is not considered to be a vitamin deficiency.

My own attitude toward using vitamins is more favorable—because I contend that arthritis is really a constitutional disorder, affecting your entire body. If you lack certain vitamins, you must correct that deficiency, or you'll hasten the onslaught of arthritic pains.

Rheumatoid arthritics, in particular, need to increase their supply of vitamins A, C and D. It is my opinion that these three vitamins are most beneficial . . . they each play an important role in restoring good health. Let's discuss these vitamins, individually.

Vitamin A favorably affects the matrix of the cartilage. It helps the cartilage to absorb proteins and enzymes.

Vitamin C contributes to the manufacture of good collagen. This enhances the tensile strength of cartilage.

Vitamin D helps to regulate the metabolism of calcium and phosphorus—an essential factor in creating strong, healthy bones and teeth.

For all arthritics, not just rheumatoid victims, I suggest that you augment your meals by taking a few special vitamins.

If you have osteoarthritis, it might be wise to take 1000 mg. of Vitamin C, with milk, at breakfast. Plus a good multi-Vitamin-Mineral supplement.

A "good" supplement is one which is made from natural or organic sources. For example, choose a vitamin combination which is manufactured from plants, fish liver oils, Brewer's yeast or torula yeast.

Stay away from vitamin supplements which have been concocted synthetically in some laboratory. Such dietary aids, created in a test-tube, are much less effective. Synthetic products do *not* have important factors like bioflavonoids and hesperidin.

If you suffer from musculoskeletal ailments, the same rules apply: try 1000 mg. of Vitamin C, and a multi-Vitamin-Mineral supplement. At breakfast, you should also ingest a 400 I.U. capsule of Vitamin E.

Vitamin E acts as an anti-oxidant and prevents the loss of oxygen from the fatty acid molecules in your bloodstream.

May I repeat that rheumatoid arthritics face the most severe problem. Their bones and cartilage have already started a "self-destruction" process. They need vitamins, urgently, to help arrest this condition.

For them, I recommend the daily intake of five key substances:

> 1000 mg. Vitamin C complex
> 400 I.U. Vitamin E complex
> 100 mg. Vitamin B complex
> 50 mg. zinc
> 50 mg. manganese

You will find more information, about vitamins, in Chapter XI. Read that Menu Section . . . it contains helpful facts, applied to all types of arthritics.

HOW I GAIN MY VITAMINS . . . FROM COD LIVER OIL!

It should be obvious, by now, that I never miss a chance to praise cod liver oil. So, naturally, you won't be surprised when I say that *this oil is a marvelous source of vitamins.*

Personally, I rely on cod liver oil to give me generous amounts of Vitamin A and Vitamin D. I have stayed healthy, for 30 years, because this oil has the ideal "balance"——the correct mix of Vitamins A and D——to nourish the human body.

What you need most, when supplying your system with these two vitamins, is a *10 to 1 ratio.* Every spoonful of cod liver oil actually contains 10 times more Vitamin A than D.

Check the label on the bottle. Almost always, it will read 4,000 USP units of Vitamin A, and then list 400 USP units of Vitamin D.

What does the term "USP units" mean? There is an international standard——a treatise on drugs and their preparation——which is called a "pharmacopeia." Therefore, cod liver oil has 4,000 units of Vitamin A, according to the United States Pharmacopeia. (In England, the ingredients are listed as BP units . . . as designated by the British Pharmacopeia.)

(Incidentally, on a bottle of cod liver oil, you may find the initials "IU" listed in regard to Vitamin E.

"IU" stands for *I*nternational *U*nits . . . a term used worldwide.)

May I make a suggestion? When you go shopping for vitamins in a store, always read the labels on each product very carefully. Be conservative in the amounts you purchase. It *is* possible to overdose your system by taking too many vitamins, too often. Seek the advice of your doctor, as to which vitamins you really require to arrest your particular ailment.

If you ingest too much Vitamin A, it can cause adverse reactions, including the loss of your hair.

Too much Vitamin D can have a toxic affect on your kidneys. So, pay close attention to your vitamin intake . . . use discretion and your own common sense.

Do you suspect that you are suffering from some form of vitamin deficiency? One way to self-diagnose such a condition is to check your own mouth.

If the tip of your tongue is often raw and red, it could be a signal that you need multi-vitamins. Is the edge of your tongue serrated? When repeated teeth imprints appear along the edges of your tongue, you undoubtedly require more B-complex vitamins.

A REASON TO SMILE . . . BETTER TEETH!

One of the happy side effects of taking cod liver oil—still another advantage—is that you will have fewer dental problems.

You can harden the enamel of your teeth, because the Vitamin D in cod liver oil contains phosphorus. This oil also causes a favorable reaction on the calcium which is already in your bloodstream. These two biochemicals (phosphorus and calcium) *when properly "oiled"* will travel more easily into the arteries of your teeth.

If you lack that Vitamin D oil, the calcium may travel *not* into your teeth, but to the surface of your bones. This could bring on osteoarthritis—you could develop bony deposits at the terminal ends of certain joints, like those in your fingers.

The appearance of your teeth and your mouth should be studied frequently. Look in your mirror . . . as a preventive measure . . . to detect certain symptoms of arthritis.

Do you have etch marks on your teeth? Is there erosion, and are your gums starting to recede? Beware, whenever you begin to have "pink toothbrush"—which could be a tell-tale sign of trouble ahead.

If you discover bleeding gums, don't ignore such a warning. That problem is often proof that you have a severe dietary deficiency. For instance, you may lack Vitamin C—and that's a necessary nutrient to improve the collagen of the cartilages in your joints.

Some highly-trained doctors and oral surgeons now agree on one fact. Like me, they have recognized the tremendous value of Vitamin C.

Personally, I shall continue to work closely with

dentists everywhere, encouraging them to study my dietary theories. I have no quarrel with the dental profession. On the contrary, dentists are showing increased interest in nutrition. Many are now urging their patients to "watch what they eat!"

Continuing my educational campaign, today I accepted an invitation to lecture before another group of enlightened dentists and oral surgeons. I shall fly to Amarillo, Texas, to keep this speaking engagement.

TMJ . . . "ARTHRITIS" OF THE JAWBONE

There is one affliction which is growing at an alarming rate. More and more people are becoming victims of *TMJ.* The initials stand for "temporomandibular joint" . . . a technical term for aches and pains in your jawbone.

The mandible is that horseshoe-shaped bone in your lower jaw which carries the lower teeth.

While I was being interviewed on a radio program, not long ago, a listener telephoned and described exactly how he hurt. He reported these symptoms: At the jawbone, near his ear, he felt something . . . as though another bone were coming down and painfully pressing his jawbone.

I advised him to see his dentist. First, he should be checked out, to determine whether he had any dental malocclusion. If the pain persisted, he could be suffering from TMJ.

In my opinion, TMJ *is* a form of arthritis. It occurs when you have poor articulation of the lower jaw.

Extensive research has been done by Dr. James C. Greenwood, Clinical Professor of Neurosurgery at the Baylor University College of Medicine. He conducted experiments using Vitamin C to combat bone pain. His findings included proof that this vitamin can stimulate the body's natural effort to repair degraded tissues and can encourage collagen formation.

HELPFUL ADVICE FROM A PROMINENT DENTIST

Among the experts I talked with recently, just before writing this book, is Emanuel Cheraskin, M.D., D.M.D., in Birmingham, Alabama. For many years, he has been nationally known as both a medical doctor and as a dentist.

Dr. Cheraskin is professor and Chairman of the Department of Oral Medicine at the University of Alabama. He advocates proper nutrition and eating habits to maintain good health. In fact, he has written several books on the importance of vitamins.

While examining the relationship between Vitamin C and arthritis, Dr. Cheraskin cites the work of Dr. B.E. Ingelmark. According to Dr. Ingelmark, *the amount of collagen—the principal portion of the white fibers of connective tissue, cartilage, and*

*bone—is directly dependent upon the amount of pro-
tein and Vitamin C available.*

For more information, helpful to arthritics, I certainly suggest that you read Dr. Cheraskin's recent
book. It is entitled *The Vitamin C Connection* (Harper
& Row, Publishers).

*Cod liver oil will reach every joint that has articu-
lar motion, including the jawbone.* To combat or to
prevent TMJ, a person should try the dietary program
outlined in this book.

———————

I wrote these past few pages—concerning teeth
and facial problems—with one purpose in mind. My
goal was to alert all arthritics . . . to make you aware
that *proper dental care is of prime importance.* Your
mouth and teeth can warn you of impending ailments,
before they spread to other parts of your body.

You should give dental hygiene a high priority in
your life. Consult a dentist, regularly. Have your teeth
cleaned, professionally. Tartar or plaque should be
removed. (These conditions, incidentally, are usually
caused by eating improperly or by a calcium imbal-
ance.)

A dentist can also detect and analyze any white
deposits or lesions on the roof of your mouth. Such
early warning signs could be a forecast of cancer.

To conclude this dental discussion, I can offer
you a very pleasant prospect for the future. From now
on you will need fewer trips to the dentist . . . if you
follow the menus and dietary rules set forth in this

book. You'll have stronger teeth, and fewer cavities!

I learn more about teeth each time I meet with Dr. Cheraskin. He and I have lectured to the same audiences. For example, we addressed a convention of the National Nutritional Foods Association. Another outstanding group, for health-conscious Americans, is NHF. To translate those initials, read on . . .

NATIONAL HEALTH FEDERATION . . . WHAT IT IS, AND WHY

Many people who read my books also read magazines on nutrition and health care. In these publications they frequently see mentioned the *National Health Federation*. During my lecture tours, I am often asked: "How important is NHF? Is it a worthwhile organization?"

I want to emphasize, here and now, that I certainly favor the work being done by the Federation. It is a group of people, nationwide, who are dedicated to achieving better health. And, most important, they are fighting for their freedom of choice . . . they want the right to select their own method of treatment when they face illness or disease.

Yes, I am proud to belong to the National Health Federation. I am a Life Member, and I actively support their goals.

When the Los Angeles Chapter of NHF celebrated their 25th Anniversary awhile back, more than

18,000 people attended the three-day event. There are 70 chapters of NHF, spread across America. The organization also maintains a legislative advocate in Washington, D.C., and he represents NHF when Congressional committees and government agencies are debating health issues.

Let me cite just two examples of battles which have been won by the Federation . . .

A decade ago, the pharmaceutical industry was promoting a law which would block the sale of *vitamins* without a doctor's prescription. NHF lobbied hard—with strong support by Senator William Proxmire of Wisconsin—and prevented the bill from being passed. Now it is still *your decision* if you want to buy vitamins to supplement your diet.

More recently, NHF has won another victory in its 28 year war with the United States Postal Service. USPS was seeking to ban the mailing of any more health books simply because the ideas in those books were not in accord with the consensus of medical opinion. Mr. Clinton Miller, the Federation's representative in Washington, made a tremendous effort to prevent this "book banning" . . . and Congress recently agreed to include several NHF amendments to Senate Bill 450. *Your freedom* to read what you wish has been protected.

I first heard about NHF way back in 1957, when I was lecturing in Washington, D.C. The Federation was founded by Mr. Fred J. Hart. He clearly stated the purpose of the organization. These are his words, his credo:

"Someone must teach the new things, someone must take the abuse, someone must be called a fraud and a quack. Then, out of it all, comes the truth to become a part of us. Thus, we receive new facts to make up our proud possession of knowledge."

Many authors, like myself, have become associated with NHF. We have taken a stand—for freedom of expression. Among the famous writers who have attended NHF conventions are Gaylord Hauser, Adelle Davis, Jack LaLanne, and many others. Carol Burnett, the television star, has also appeared and has spoken out in support of the Federation.

Personally, I have lectured before NHF groups from coast to coast . . . at some 30 events, ranging from Seattle to Tucson, from Chicago to Orlando, Florida.

I shall continue to serve the Federation, whenever I'm asked, throughout my lifetime.

———————

When I began writing this chapter, my primary purpose was to warn you about the dangers of acidity. I denounced the drinking of citrus fruit juices, and showed you how citric acid can destroy your pH level.

Now, in conclusion, let me cite an even worse threat. Carbonated cola drinks are still manufactured with *phosphoric acid* as an active ingredient. Today, to confirm this fact, I visited the Chemistry Department at UCLA. University chemists took a popular brand of soda pop—a cola drink—and tested it.

The research scientists used a Corning pH meter, Model 5, and determined an indisputable fact: The pH of the cola drink is 2.2. More negative than pure lemon juice!

Remember, your saliva has a pH rating of 7. Subtract the 2.2 rating of the cola drink from 7. That leaves a deplorable 4.8 of acid which is never neutralized in your mouth. When you gulp down the bottle of soda pop, all that acid has to be buffered by your digestive system and organs.

With this graphic proof—and real condemnation—I'll end my acid remarks.

CHAPTER X

Proper Timing . . . When To Consume Foods And Liquids

Let's assume that you have selected healthful foods, and you are following the recommended menus. You feel content . . . because you are confident that you have a "balanced" diet.

Sorry. You may be wrong. Many people wreck the "balance" in their diet—by drinking the wrong liquids at mealtime. If you consume certain beverages with your meals, you diminish the nutritional value of all your foods.

In this chapter, I won't be repeating my severe criticism of soda pop. You already know how I detest carbonated drinks and acidic juices. Now, I want to discuss some problems related to drinking *water*. Then, I'll give you good news on the benefits of *milk*.

Timing is crucial. There is a proper sequence for eating foods . . . and important rules as to when you should drink liquids. For example, you should never drink a glass of water at mealtime to "wash down" healthy morsels of food.

You want to gain the maximum "lubricating" power—from the edible oils contained in that food. Don't congeal those oils, in your stomach, by drinking ice-cubed water. It's an old adage, but it still holds true: Oil and water don't mix!

110

How can anyone be "against" ordinary drinking water? I assure you, I am *not* anti-water. The truth is, I recommend that you drink two glasses of water every morning, before breakfast. (See the Menus, in Chapter XI.)

Water, preferably warm, can serve as a mild laxative and will help flush your kidneys. It also contains minerals and other helpful properties.

My main suggestion is that you drink water when your stomach is empty. Consume this liquid early in the morning, or four hours after dinner, just before you retire at night.

I do not recommend distilled water. But I am in favor of bottled spring water—that's best of all!

For years, many Americans have been brainwashed into thinking that everybody needs 8 glasses of water per day in order to stay healthy. I believe that is sheer nonsense. If you are eating 2,200 calories per day, your body requires 6½ glasses of *some kind of fluid.* It can come from milk, from soup, from eating an apple or a piece of celery. Fluids are available, each day, from many sources.

If you inundate the grass on your front lawn with too much water, the grass becomes waterlogged and dies. Don't "waterlog" yourself with too many glassfuls of various liquids. It's unnecessary.

Using ice cubes in your beverages is the most grievous mistake anyone can make. Drinking icy liquids with your meals, is a common error. During digestion, your dietary oils will quickly congeal . . . their value is literally lost.

During my lectures, I have sometimes compared

the human digestive system with the mechanical parts of an automobile . . .

Your family car has three separate compartments. You provide water for the water pump. You supply oil for the oil pump. And you place gasoline in the tank.

At no time do you "mix" these liquids. Nobody adds water to the gasoline tank or to the compartment meant for oil.

The human machine has only two pumps. First, there's the heart——which pumps blood. And the second vessel is the stomach——which *can* pump dietary oils to various points throughout your body.

However, *the stomach is unable to pump properly if you are drinking water and other oil-free liquids with your meals.*

THE IMPORTANCE OF WAITING . . . BEFORE YOU DRINK LIQUIDS

After eating a meal, I maintain that a person should fast for approximately four hours before you drink any oil-free liquid.

Give your stomach *time* to act.

The lacteals and villi in your gastro-intestinal tract must also have adequate time to assimilate your foods. The process of assimilation, vitally important to all arthritics, is fully described on page 31.

The idea of allowing your food to be absorbed——before you cram new foods or liquids into your stomach—is not just a Dale Alexander hypothesis. I have substantial evidence, gathered from *The Annals of Internal Medicine,* which supports this theory.

A published report, more than 40 years ago, addressed this same topic. An article appeared (in April of 1941) giving credence to the habit of *post-absorptive fasting.* The author was Dr. Irvine Page, who later became world-renowned for his research on cholesterol.

Dr. Page recommended fasting between meals, to help stabilize cholesterol levels. He gained prominence for his work at the Cleveland Clinic. Now retired, Dr. Page lives in Hyannisport, Massachusetts. I telephoned him, recently, and commended him for his pioneering research related to food and proper eating habits.

I might add that I am against "snack foods" if they are consumed between meals. Give your stomach at least four hours to digest and assimilate a meal. That's my interpretation of post-absorptive fasting.

MILK . . . YOUR MOST VALUABLE ALLY AMONG ALL LIQUIDS

Milk has been called "the perfect food"—and I agree that it has fine qualities. Each glass of milk gives you calcium, Vitamins A and D, and it even contains a percentage of butter fat.

Because milk, itself, is an oil-bearing liquid, this makes it compatible with the *assimilation* we are trying to achieve inside our bodies.

While being digested, milk is a liquid with low surface tension—able to assist in transporting oil globules. It can help your dietary oils to by-pass your liver, so they can be carried more readily to your lymphatic system.

For all these reasons, I now tell arthritics to mix their cod liver oil with milk. This represents a change from the recommendations I made in my first book. I originally suggested that you prepare a daily mixture made with orange juice and cod liver oil. You can still employ that method . . . but I now offer you the option of using milk, for equally healthful results.

After much research, to find an alternative for orange juice, I found that milk had many advantages. (Another factor involved was that too many people were starting to use *the wrong kind* of orange juice. In recent years, frozen concentrates of orange juice were invented. Unfortunately, some of my readers were taking cans of concentrate from their refrigerators. They would then add water—a real sin!—to make their orange juice.)

If you prefer the taste of orange juice to milk, then just make sure that you use fresh fruit, squeezed by hand. Follow the specific rules on pages 117–119.

At times, I have been asked whether drinking milk will lead to a cholesterol problem. My answer is an emphatic "No!"

We have been subjected to "a cholesterol

scare''—a nationwide alarm which is without foundation. In my opinion, some very vocal cardiologists spoke too hastily and they frightened millions of people. "Take the milk—and the butter and eggs—out of your diet!" This loud warning temporarily revised the eating habits of too many Americans.

Additional research is now causing this trend to be reversed. I hope for a return to normalcy.

Become a milk drinker. If you want to avoid a heart attack, or a stroke, milk can improve the quality of your arteries. You can add more elasticity to your arteries . . . so they won't "balloon out" and explode, like a flat tire. Why suffer an aneurysm or a stroke?

For victims of arthritis, may I emphasize that I am recommending whole milk. Not skim milk, nor chocolate milk, nor canned milk.

Stay with whole milk . . . either raw certified, homogenized, or pasteurized.

TIMING TIPS . . . FOR "NIGHT PEOPLE" AND LATE WORKERS

Your occupation may force you to eat your meals at irregular hours. If you work the "swing shift" at night, you are not in the habit of having breakfast at 7 a.m. or lunch at noon.

Therefore, perhaps I should give some special suggestions—a different timetable for arthritics who do most of their eating at night. When you read the menus, in the next Chapter, you can substitute hours of your own choice for all three daily meals.

Just remember the principle of post-absorptive fasting. Wait four hours after each meal before you drink water. (Or, you can drink a glass of water ten minutes before any meal. The main requisite is to consume liquids when your stomach is empty . . . as near empty as possible.)

Adjust your taking of cod liver oil based on this same "empty stomach" approach.

Starting today, enjoy eating! In the pages just ahead, you'll find many delicious meals and recipes.

COD LIVER OIL SCHEDULE

Two principal points must work in harmony.

The Dietary regimen must serve as insurance to guarantee the benefits to be derived from sustained use of Cod Liver Oil.

Take the Cod Liver Oil mixture for six months. Then take it once or twice a week for your lifetime.

Earwax checked by a cotton covered Q-tip® should register yellow, soft, and pasty.

If necessary take an additional six months

COD LIVER OIL
IS YOUR KEY
WEAPON

PLAN 1—TO MIX COD LIVER OIL WITH MILK . . .

First, you'll need to have a tablespoon and a small, four-ounce jar. A baby food jar, with a screw top, will do just fine.

Place two tablespoons of whole milk into the jar. The milk can be brought directly from the refrigerator.

Next, add one tablespoon of pure cod liver oil. *Shake vigorously*, for approximately 10 seconds. Notice the oil globules . . . you are emulsifying the oil, temporarily, before you ingest it. The whole milk renders the oil almost tasteless. Now, drink this mixture immediately—on an empty stomach—at the time indicated in the Menus on pages 121 thru 129. Also, consult the drawing on the next page.

PLAN 2—TO MIX COD LIVER OIL & ORANGE JUICE . . .

Using a tablespoon and the same type of jar as the one described above, you can employ orange juice as the emulsifier.

I recommend that you *hand-squeeze* half an orange, to obtain approximately two tablespoons of juice to place into the jar. (You want no pulp to hinder assimilation.)

Now, add one tablespoonful of cod liver oil. Remember, for Plan 1 or Plan 2, you can choose oil that is plain, mint, or cherry flavored. Shake the mixture, briskly, for five to ten seconds. When it becomes frothy, drink it promptly. Orange concentrates are not to be used, only fresh fruit. Turn this page, to learn the Plan 2 drinking timetable.

COD LIVER OIL WITH MILK • PLAN I

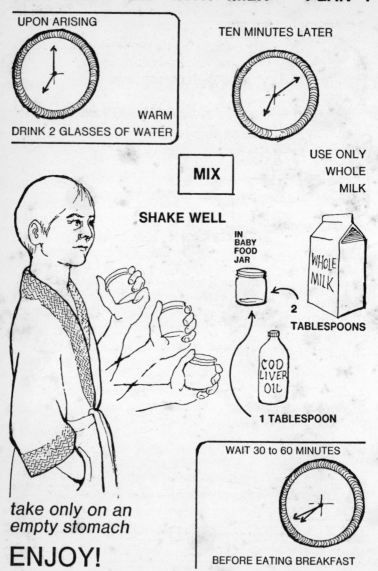

UPON ARISING

WARM
DRINK 2 GLASSES OF WATER

TEN MINUTES LATER

MIX

USE ONLY
WHOLE
MILK

SHAKE WELL

IN
BABY
FOOD
JAR

WHOLE
MILK

2
TABLESPOONS

COD
LIVER
OIL

1 TABLESPOON

*take only on an
empty stomach*

ENJOY!

WAIT 30 to 60 MINUTES

BEFORE EATING BREAKFAST

COD LIVER OIL WITH ORANGE JUICE •
PLAN II

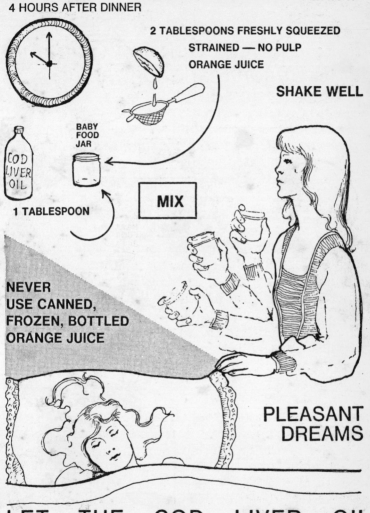

4 HOURS AFTER DINNER

2 TABLESPOONS FRESHLY SQUEEZED
STRAINED — NO PULP
ORANGE JUICE

SHAKE WELL

COD LIVER OIL

BABY FOOD JAR

MIX

1 TABLESPOON

NEVER
USE CANNED,
FROZEN, BOTTLED
ORANGE JUICE

PLEASANT
DREAMS

LET THE COD LIVER OIL
WORK WHILE YOU SLEEP

CHAPTER XI

Menus . . . A Detailed Guide of Recommended Menus

To recover from arthritis—to get well and stay well—you will need to concentrate and do some planning. Menu planning.

You must remember to avoid certain foods and beverages which are highly acidic . . . but that's only half the battle. It is equally important that you "balance" your diet . . . by eating sufficient quantities of good food each day. In other words, you must plan ahead. Make a list of meals, for an entire week. You can include a variety of tasty dishes, and still be eating your way toward better health.

For your guidance, I have compiled a dietary schedule based on very wholesome foods. My suggestions for mealtime are easy to follow.

You may be pleasantly surprised by the menus I offer in these next few pages. Eating should always be an enjoyable experience. These meals—recommended for arthritics—will be appealing to your palate. They are flavorsome *and* nutritious.

Notice that I have designed three complete sets of menus. They are arranged on a day-by-day basis—a typical guide for an entire week. Depending on the type of arthritis which applies to you, and how severe your affliction may be, you can select the correct group of meals. Bon appetit!

MENUS FOR THOSE WITH OSTEOARTHRITIS

MONDAY

UPON ARISING
7 a.m. ....2 glasses of water
(preferably warm)
7:10 a.m. ....Cod Liver Oil Mixture
7:40 a.m. ....Breakfast

BREAKFAST
Whole grain cereal ..1 cup
Bran ....2 tbsp.
Whole milk (with ce-
real).....................4 oz.
Prunes.....................6 or 8
Whole milk ....4 oz.

LUNCH
Mixed green salad
Omelette
Whole milk ....8 oz.

DINNER
Green salad
Chicken casserole
Whole grain noodles
Fresh fruit cup
Whole milk ....8 oz.

TUESDAY

UPON ARISING
7 a.m. ....2 glasses of water
(preferably warm)
7:10 a.m. ....Cod Liver Oil Mixture
7:40 a.m. ....Breakfast

BREAKFAST
Poached or soft-boiled eggs................. 2
Whole wheat toast
Butter .... 1 pat
Whole milk .... 8 oz.

LUNCH
Bran muffin
Butter ....1 pat
Cottage cheese soup
Green salad
Whole milk ....8 oz.

DINNER
Broiled steak
Small green salad
Potato strips (See Recipe, Page 132)
Carrots amd zucchini (steamed)
Whole milk ....8 oz.

WEDNESDAY

UPON ARISING
7 a.m. ....2 glasses of water
(preferably warm)
7:10 a.m. ....Cod Liver Oil Mixture
7:40 a.m. ....Breakfast

BREAKFAST
Fresh fruit cup
Cheese and parsley omelette
Whole grain toast ....1 slice
Butter and Honey
Whole milk ....8 oz.

LUNCH
Chicken salad
Whole grain crackers
Sliced peaches or
fresh fruit (in season)
Whole milk ....8 oz.

DINNER
Spinach salad
Vegetarian dinner
Silky's cake ....small slice
(See Recipe, Page 136)
Whole milk ....8 oz.

Menus . . . A Detailed Guide of Recommended Menus

THURSDAY

UPON ARISING
7 a.m. ....2 glasses of water
(preferably warm)
7:10 a.m. ....Cod Liver Oil Mixture
7:40 a.m. ....Breakfast

BREAKFAST
Cooked rolled oats ..1 cup
Bran ....2 tbsp.
Whole milk ....2 oz.
Prunes ....6 or 8
Whole milk ....6 oz.

LUNCH
Poached eggs on
toast 2
Mixed green salad
Whole milk ....8 oz.

DINNER
Broiled hamburger melt
Baked potato ....1 medium
Brussels sprouts .....½ cup
Grated carrot salad ..½ cup
Whole milk ....8 oz.

FRIDAY

UPON ARISING
7 a.m. ....2 glasses of water
(preferably warm)
7:10 a.m. ....Cod Liver Oil Mixture
7:40 a.m. ....Breakfast

BREAKFAST
Granola cereal ....1 cup
Bran ....2 tbsp.
Whole milk ....4 oz.
Berries and plain whole yogurt
Whole milk ....4 oz.

LUNCH
Tuna sandwich on 7-grain bread
Green salad
Whole milk ....8 oz.

DINNER
Gazpacho
Broiled halibut and steamed carrots
Fresh fruit cup
Carob cookie
Whole milk ....8 oz.

SATURDAY

UPON ARISING
7 a.m. ....2 glasses of water
(preferably warm)
7:10 a.m. ....Cod Liver Oil Mixture
7:40 a.m. ....Breakfast

BREAKFAST
Buckwheat pancakes
Freckled banana and whole yogurt
Whole milk ....8 oz.

LUNCH
Hamburger patty on sesame roll
Green salad
Whole milk ....8 oz.

DINNER
Chicken casserole with
Brown rice
Silky's cake
Whole milk ....8 oz.

SUNDAY

UPON ARISING
7 a.m. ....2 glasses of water
(preferably warm)
7:10 a.m. ....Cod Liver Oil Mixture
7:40 a.m. ....Breakfast

BREAKFAST
Choice of fruit
Corn or bran muffins
Canadian bacon or lean ham
Eggs........................2
Whole milk ....8 oz.

LUNCH
Mixed green salad
Corn tortilla with
Cheddar cheese (in broiler
until cheese melts)
Whole milk ....8 oz.

DINNER
Oriental vegetables over brown rice
Whole almonds and chicken on top
Tapioca pudding .....1 cup
Whole milk ....8 oz.

The meals which I have outlined—for anyone with osteoarthritis—are highly nutritious. As long as you *chew* the foods properly to gain their full value.

More than a few senior citizens, with arthritis, have asked me what they should do if they have trouble in chewing. Sometimes they have ill-fitting dentures.

Here's one suggestion: a raw salad can be mixed in a blender with a little milk. Add seasoning or salad dressing. *Drink* your salad *slowly*.

Cooked vegetables, still firm, can be homogenized in a blender with some milk. Add a bit of seasoning, as desired. As another variation, just by adding more milk, you create a delicious soup.

If your teeth present no problem, then forge ahead happily, and try these menus.

Chew. Mix your saliva with whatever you eat. *Chewing* your food adds *ptyalin* for better digestion. Ptyalin in your saliva is an enzyme that converts starch into various dextrins and maltose.

MENUS FOR THOSE WITH RHEUMATOID ARTHRITIS

MONDAY

UPON ARISING
7 a.m. ....2 glasses of water
(preferably warm)
7:10 a.m. ....Cod Liver Oil Mixture
7:40 a.m. ....Breakfast

BREAKFAST
Special Health Drink
(See Formula on page 126)

Vitamin Supplements
(At breakfast time,
daily, if you have
rheumatoid arthritis,
you should also take
the vitamin supplements
listed on Page 99.)

LUNCH
Cottage cheese ....½ cup
Fresh fruit slices
Date nut bread
Cream cheese ....1 tbsp.
Whole milk ....8 oz.

DINNER
Broiled lamb chops ..2 small
Baked yam
Broccoli ....½ cup
Fluffed Rice Pudding
(See Recipe, Page 137)
Whole milk ....8 oz.

TUESDAY

UPON ARISING
7 a.m. ....2 glasses of water
(preferably warm)
7:10 a.m. ....Cod Liver Oil Mixture
7:40 a.m. ....Breakfast

BREAKFAST
Special Health Drink
(Same as Monday Breakfast)

Vitamin Supplements
(Same as Monday)

LUNCH
Whole grain English muffin (toasted)
Cheddar or Jack
cheese ....1 slice
Melon ....¼
Whole Milk ....8 oz.

DINNER
Clear soup ....1 cup
Oriental Vegetable Delight
(See Recipe, Page 138)
Whole milk ....8 oz.

WEDNESDAY

UPON ARISING
7 a.m. ....2 glasses of water
(preferably warm)
7:10 a.m. ....Cod Liver Oil Mixture
7:40 a.m. ....Breakfast

BREAKFAST
Special Health Drink
Vitamin Supplements

LUNCH
Fresh fruit salad
Bran mufflin 1
Butter ....1 pat
Whole milk ....8 oz.

DINNER
Tossed green salad
Broiled hamburger steak
Baked potato ....1 small
Swiss chard ....1 cup
Carrot yogurt cake ...1 slice
Whole milk ....8 oz.

Menus . . . A Detailed Guide of Recommended Menus

THURSDAY

UPON ARISING
7 a.m. ....2 glasses of water
(preferably warm)
7:10 a.m. ....Cod Liver Oil Mixture
7:40 a.m. ....Breakfast

BREAKFAST
Special Health Drink

Vitamin Supplements

LUNCH
Toss and fluff spinach salad
Hot corn bread
Butter ....1 pat
Whole milk ....8 oz.

DINNER
Spinach salad
Baked chicken casserole
Whole grain noodles ½ cup
String beans ....½ cup
Whole milk ....8 oz.

FRIDAY

UPON ARISING
7 a.m. ....2 glasses of water
(preferably warm)
7:10 a.m. ....Cod Liver Oil Mixture
7:40 a.m. ....Breakfast

BREAKFAST
Special Health Drink

Vitamin Supplements

LUNCH
Deviled egg sandwich
Carrot and celery sticks
Corn chips ....½ cup
Slice of pineapple
Whole milk ....8 oz.

DINNER
Mixed green salad
Broiled fish or steak
Potato strips
Carrots and peas.....½ cup
Silky's cake ....small piece
(See Recipe, Page 136)
Whole milk ....8 oz.

SATURDAY

UPON ARISING
7 a.m. ....2 glasses of water
(preferably warm)
7:10 a.m. ....Cod Liver Oil Mixture
7:40 a.m. ....Breakfast

BREAKFAST
Special Health Drink

Vitamin Supplements

LUNCH
Cottage cheese vegetable soup
Hot corn bread........1 square
Butter ....1 pat
Honey ....1 tbsp.
Whole milk ....8 oz.

DINNER
Mixed green salad
Broiled calves' liver or other meat
Corn on the cob
Carrot yogurt cake
Whole milk ....8 oz.

SUNDAY

UPON ARISING

7 a.m. ....2 glasses of water
(preferably warm)
7:10 a.m. ....Cod Liver Oil Mixture
7:40 a.m. ....Breakfast

BREAKFAST

Special Health Drink

Vitamin Supplements

LUNCH

Mixed vegetable salad
Corn tortilla, topped
with Jack or
cheddar cheese
(broil until cheese melts)
Whole milk ....8 oz.

DINNER

Chicken broth ....1 cup
Broiled chicken
Buckwheat(Kasha)..1 cup
Brussels sprouts
Carrot yogurt cake ..1 slice
Whole milk ....8 oz.

In the group of menus you have just read, please note that I ask you to augment these foods by taking vitamin supplements. (See the list on page 99.)

For victims of rheumatoid arthritis, especially, the formula published below could be most beneficial.

I recommend that you take this drink daily, for at least six months. This is how you make it:

SPECIAL HEALTH DRINK

1 tsp. Chia seed
1 tsp. Sunflower seeds
6 oz. whole milk

Soak seeds for 15 minutes in . . .

1 fertile egg
1 tbsp. soybean or sunflower oil
1 tbsp. Acidophilus Culture
Pinch of sea kelp powder
½ tsp. of rose hips powder
1 tsp. Brewer's or torula yeast
1 tsp. lecithin
1 tsp. malted coconut
1 freckled banana

Blend in a blender and drink.

It's a complete breakfast!

MENUS FOR THOSE WITH MUSCULOSKELETAL ARTHRITIS

If you have musculoskeletal problems (some examples are: tendinitis, myositis, sciatica rheumatism, bursitis, fibrositis, neuritis, shin splints, etc.) I recommend the following meals:

MONDAY

UPON ARISING
7 a.m. ....2 glasses of water (preferably warm)
7:10 a.m. ....Cod Liver Oil Mixture
7:40 a.m. ....Breakfast

BREAKFAST
Whole grain cereal...1 cup
Bran ....2 tbsp.
Whole milk (with cereal) 4 oz.
Prunes....................6 or 8
Whole milk ....4 oz.

LUNCH
Mixed green salad
Omelette ....2 eggs
Whole milk ....8 oz.

DINNER
Waldorf salad
(apples, celery, nuts, mayonnaise)
Leg of lamb..............2 slices
Carrots and peas.....1 cup
Tapioca pudding .....½ cup
Whole milk ....8 oz.

TUESDAY

UPON ARISING
7 a.m. ....2 glasses of water (preferably warm)
7:10 a.m. ....Cod Liver Oil Mixture
7:40 a.m. ....Breakfast

BREAKFAST
Poached eggs.........2
Whole wheat toast...1 slice
Whole yogurt...........½ cup
Prunes....................6
Whole milk ....8 oz.

LUNCH
Tossed green salad
Grilled cheese sandwich
Apple
Whole milk ....8 oz.

DINNER
Vegetable soup ....6 oz.
Cheese enchilada....2
Celery and carrot stix
Brown rice ....½ cup
Whole milk ....8 oz.

WEDNESDAY

UPON ARISING
7 a.m. ....2 glasses of water (preferably warm)
7:10 a.m. ....Cod Liver Oil Mixture
7:40 a.m. ....Breakfast

BREAKFAST
Granola cereal ....½ cup
Raw wheat germ .....2 tbsp.
Plain whole yogurt...4 oz.
Sliced fresh fruit
Whole milk ....8 oz.

LUNCH
Mixed green salad
Brisket of beef ....1 slice
Cookie 1
Whole milk ....8 oz.

DINNER
Lima bean soup.......½ cup
Broiled calves' liver or steak
Baked yam..............1 small
String beans ....½ cup
Sliced fruit ....½ cup
Whole milk ....8 oz.

Menus . . . A Detailed Guide of Recommended Menus

THURSDAY

UPON ARISING
7 a.m. ....2 glasses of water
(preferably warm)
7:10 a.m. ....Cod Liver Oil Mixture
7:40 a.m. ....Breakfast

BREAKFAST
Special Health Drink
(See Formula on Page 126)

Vitamin Supplements
(Listed on Page 99)

LUNCH
Tuna sandwich on whole grain bread
Green Romaine lettuce and tomato
Pear
Whole milk ....8 oz.

DINNER
Green salad with tomato
Roast pork ....2 slices
Baked potato ....1 small
Asparagus...............4 spears
Whole yogurt and strawberries
Whole milk ....8 oz.

FRIDAY

UPON ARISING
7 a.m. ....2 glasses of water
(preferably warm)
7:10 a.m. ....Cod Liver Oil Mixture
7:40 a.m. ....Breakfast

BREAKFAST
Whole grain hot cereal
Raw wheat germ .....2 tbsp.
Whole milk (on ce-
real)....................2 oz.
Whole yogurt and prunes
Whole milk ....6 oz.

LUNCH
Sliced cold meat
(ham, pork, or veal)
Tossed green salad
Cookie
Whole milk ....8 oz.

DINNER
Shrimp cocktail
Broiled lobster
Potato strips
Stewed tomato ....½ cup
Green beans ....½ cup
Silky's cake ....1 slice
Whole milk ....8 oz.

SATURDAY

UPON ARISING
7 a.m. ....2 glasses of water
(preferably warm)
7:10 a.m. ....Cod Liver Oil Mixture
7:40 a.m. ....Breakfast

BREAKFAST
Choice of fresh fruit
Bran or corn muffin and butter
Scrambled eggs 2
Lean ham or Canadian bacon
Whole milk ....8 oz.

LUNCH
Chicken salad
Corn bread..............1 square
Butter ....1 pad
Melon ....¼

DINNER
Vegetable soup
Cheese enchilada....2
Celery and carrot stix
Brown rice ....½ cup
Fresh fruit cup
Whole milk ....8 oz.

SUNDAY

UPON ARISING
7 a.m. ....2 glasses of water
                   (preferably warm)
7:10 a.m. ....Cod Liver Oil Mixture
7:40 a.m. ....Breakfast

BREAKFAST
Fresh fruit cup
Buckwheat pancakes with
Butter and honey
Whole milk ....8 oz.

LUNCH
Date nut bread (whole grain)
Cream cheese.........1 tbsp.
Fruit salad
Whole milk ....8 oz.

DINNER
Spinach salad
Broiled chicken
Potato strips
String beans ....½ cup
Carrot yogurt cake...1 slice
Whole milk ....8 oz.

DINING IN RESTAURANTS . . . SOME CAUTIOUS REMINDERS

We all have a favorite restaurant, a place we like to go on special occasions. "Dining out" is a joy . . . so, once in awhile, let someone else serve you. Let them do the dishes.

All I ask is that you use some discretion when you choose a restaurant. Does the cafe or dining room offer an abundance of natural foods? Inquire whether their menu includes plenty of unprocessed, unsprayed foods.

Too many restaurants and "fast food" places rely very heavily on the use of flavor enhancers, emulsifiers, and preservative sprays.

Some restaurateurs have been spraying sodium bisulfite on fresh fruits, vegetables, shrimp, chicken, etc. The average citizen, in America, consumes 2 to 3 milligrams of sulfites each day. Where "spraying" occurs, ingesting restaurant salads and vegetables can give a person 20 to 100 milligrams in one restaurant meal!

I maintain that the menus and dietary rules published in this Chapter can do much to alleviate pain for millions of people who already have arthritis. Equally important, this nutritional program is also designed for a healthy person—as a method to help *prevent* arthritic ailments.

On the topic of preventing illness, I recently read a report which contained several very intelligent comments made by Dr. Williard Gaylen, President of the Hastings Institute in New York. Attributed to him were these wise statements:

"If a person followed several common sense rules for a healthy lifestyle (like proper diet, regular exercise, not smoking, routine relaxation, good hygiene, etc.) the health benefits derived would be much greater than that achieved through all the fancy medical technology of the last century.

Unfortunately, most people do not take *preventive medicine* seriously enough and prefer to live with their vices in the hope of being "saved" by medical research.

It is equally unfortunate that, from the viewpoint of the medical profession, there is no profit in prevention."

Well said, Dr. Gaylen! I agree, totally. May I add that, in my opinion, the most important factor to stave off illness is a person's diet. To summarize, the best weapon can be described in just four words: Nutrition and Common Sense.

A ROUND-UP OF "REAL GOOD" RECIPES

Meals can be sheer enjoyment . . . and they become supreme if the person who does the cooking happens to know a few "extra special" recipes.

Quite often, whenever I eat a very appetizing main course or dessert, I ask for the recipe. I check the ingredients—to make sure they are healthful—and then I add that recipe to my prized collection.

Recipes are to save and savor. So, let me share some of my favorites with you.

Baked Chicken Casserole

1 large onion, diced
1 can of tomato sauce

¼ pound of mushrooms, sliced
1 frying chicken, cut up

Combine the onion, mushrooms and tomato sauce. Spread one-half of the mixture on an 8 x 14-inch Pyrex baking dish. Place chicken pieces on top of this sauce. Then, cover the chicken with the rest of the tomato mixture. Sprinkle with seasoning. Bake at 325 degrees, covered with foil, for one hour. Remove the foil. Bake again, for another half-hour. *Serves 4.*

Chili Beans Supreme
"Where's the beef?" • With the beans!

1 pound of pink or red beans
1 pound can of tomato purée
½ pound of ground beef
1 large onion, diced
1 clove of garlic, chopped
1 red onion, diced, for garnish

parsley
½ tsp. thyme
½ tsp. oregano
1 tsp. chili powder
1 tsp. sea salt

Cover the beans with water, in a 2-quart pan, and soak overnight. Next day, add the tomato purée and simmer for one hour. Quickly, fry the ground beef, without using fat, until the beef loses the raw color. Keep stirring the beef constantly . . . then add it to the beans. In the same pan, sauté the diced onion, until lightly browned. Add the onion to the beans. Add garlic, herbs and seasoning. Next, cook the entire mixture for four hours, or until the beans are tender. Stir, occasionally. Serve with chopped red onions. *Serves 6.*

Toasted Potato Strips

These ''strips'' are a treat. Instead of French fries, try this substitute . . . Cut a whole potato in half, length-wise. Cut each half, in half again, length-wise. Do it once more, and now you'll have strips about the size of French fries. Place the pieces, skin side down, on the tray of a toaster oven. Bake (at 400 degrees F.) for about 15 minutes—or more—until they are well browned. Toast the potatoes, do not fry them. This way, there's no fat and no salt, yet the result is delicious!

Baked Fish • Red Snapper

2 carrots, sliced	1 lb. of red snapper (filleted)
2 potatoes, diced	1 onion, diced
½ lb. of string beans, halved	¼ lb. of mushrooms, sliced
1 zucchini squash, sliced	1 tbsp. of butter
2 tbsp. of water	Seasoning of your choice

Pre-cook the carrots, potatoes, string beans and zucchini in water. Add seasoning. When the vegetables are crisp and tender, spread them on a casserole, along with the liquid from the vegetables. Sauté the onion and the mushrooms in butter, until lightly browned. Spread them over the vegetables. Next, take thin slices of the fish and place them over the vegetables. Sprinkle seasoning on the fish. Broil until the fish turns white— which takes approximately 10 to 15 minutes. The fish tastes best when it is barely cooked. You may substitute other types of fish—like sea bass, whitefish, or flounder. *Serves 4.*

Mash and Smash Tuna Salad

6 hard-boiled eggs	½ red onion, diced
1 can tuna	Hickory-smoked enzyme seasoning
15 sprigs of parsley, chopped	oregano
3 tbsp. of mayonnaise	alfalfa sprouts

1 oz. Galliano liqueur (optional)

Mash and smash the eggs, with a wide fork. Mix in the two tablespoons of mayonnaise. Add the parsley, sprinkle with seasoning. Mash and smash the entire mixture again. Add the onion, half of the tuna, and more seasoning. Mash and smash. Finally, add a sprinkling of the alfalfa sprouts. Serve on slices of whole grain bread, using a teaspoonful of mayonnaise as a spread. (As an optional extra, for a little more "smash" in the salad, you can also add one ounce of Galliano liqueur.) *Serves 4.*

Cheese Enchiladas

Sauce Ingredients:
1 can (15 oz.) of tomato sauce
½ cup of water
2 tbsp. chili powder
1 tsp. cumin
½ tsp. turmeric

Filling Ingredients:
2 medium onions, chopped
4 oz. of ripe olives, chopped
2 tbsp. cold pressed oil
1 lb. of Jack cheese
½ lb. of cheddar cheese
Grated American cheese

1 dozen corn tortillas

Mix the sauce ingredients in a medium-sized frying pan. Let them simmer, while you prepare the tortilla filling. To prepare the filling, sauté the chopped onions in the oil. Set the onions aside. Cut each of the cheeses into 12 strips that will easily fit into the rolled tortillas.

Dip one tortilla into the heated sauce. Then, in the middle of the tortilla, place a heaping tablespoonful of the olive-onion mixture——plus a strip of each of the two cheeses.

Roll the tortilla around the filling, and place in an 8 x 10-inch baking pan. Continue this process until all the tortillas are rolled and filled. Pour the remaining sauce over the rolled tortillas. Top with grated cheese. Cover with foil. Bake at 350 degrees, for approximately 30 minutes——or until the cheese melts and the sauce is bubbly. The enchiladas can be assembled in the morning, and then baked just before serving. These enchiladas freeze well, for reheating later.

(In all these recipes, where I refer to "oil" as an ingredient, I mean cold pressed oil. Oils which have not been cold pressed have been "heated" during processing to prolong their shelf life . . . and some of the beneficial fatty acids have been lost.)

Chicken Liver Sauté

1 lb. of chicken livers	1 onion, diced
¼ lb. of mushrooms, diced	1 pat of butter

Sauté the diced onion in butter. Add the mushrooms. When lightly browned, push the onions and mushrooms aside in the pan, and add the chicken livers. Turn the livers, browning them lightly, until they lose the raw look. Then, mix the liver and onions together. Cut into one piece of liver to see if it is done on the inside. If it looks too raw, cook some more . . . but do not overcook. This delectable dish can be served with a baked potato for dinner—or, with scrambled eggs, for breakfast. *Serves 4.*

Toss & Fluff Spinach Salad

1 bunch of spinach, chopped	3 tbsp. cold pressed oil
6 hard-boiled eggs	Hickory-smoked enzyme seasoning
(mashed with a fork)	oregano
bacon bits (optional)	1 tsp. of cider vinegar

Place half of the oil at the bottom of a mixing bowl. Use only the greenest fresh spinach . . . and be sure it is dry. Sprinkle on the seasoning. Add the eggs, plus some more seasoning. Add the diced onion. Mix and churn. Then, add the bacon bits and the rest of the oil. Toss and fluff as you go along, sprinkling in the rest of the seasoning. *Serves 4.*

Gazpacho

5 ripe tomatoes	3 tbsp. cold pressed oil
2 tsp. vinegar	1 tsp. seasoning mix
1 cup of tomato juice	1 small onion, chopped

Blend for two minutes in a blender. Chill, in a soup tureen. If you wish, you might also add some chopped cucumber—plus additional onion and green pepper. You could add some croutons, and garnish with chopped parsley. *Serves 5.*

Zesty Fresh Fruit Salad

½ cup of yogurt	Assorted fruit
¼ cup of cottage cheese	2 tbsp. of honey

Menus . . . A Detailed Guide of Recommended Menus

Your choice of fresh fruits can include peaches, pears, apricots, mango, papaya, persimmon, apples, etc. Cut the fruit into slices or chunks. Combine the yogurt and cottage cheese and honey. Embellish your salad by pouring this mixture over the fruit.

Cottage Cheese Vegetable Soup

1 whole potato, unpeeled	1 large carrot, sliced
1 whole yam, unpeeled	2 stalks of celery, sliced
1 small onion, diced	1 large tomato
2 scoops, cottage cheese	(cut into wedges)

Cover all the ingredients, except the cottage cheese, with water. Cook slowly, in a covered pan, until tender. Remove potato and yam. Peel and dice them, then return them to the soup. Add mixed seasoning to taste. Serve in soup bowls, over a scoop of cottage cheese. Sprinkle with chopped parsley. *Serves 2.*

Creative Soup

4 soup bones	4 cups of water
½ cup legumes	1 onion
2 carrots	3 stalks of celery
1 tomato	

Boil the bones in water, until a heavy foam forms on top. Lower the heat, and skim the soup. Add the legumes. Or, if you wish, you can create pea soup—by adding split peas. As another variation, you can make bean soup—by using lima beans or lentils. If you like a thicker soup, use more legumes. Next, add the vegetables, and cook slowly, until tender. The larger the beans, the longer it takes to cook. Season to taste. Garnish with chopped parsley. You can also purée this soup. *Serves 4.*

Saucy Salad Dressing

2 tbsp. vinegar	2 tbsp. seasoning mix
2 tbsp. honey	1 cup of cold pressed oil

Place vinegar, honey and seasoning mix in a pint bottle. Set the bottle in a bowl of hot water, until the honey melts. Shake the bottle vigorously. Add the oil, a little at a time, shaking the bottle after each addition. Refrigerate. Just before serving, on a salad, shake the dressing again, for maximum taste appeal.

Green Garnish Salad Dressing

⅔ cup of buttermilk
½ cup of cottage cheese
¼ tsp. tarragon

3 tbsp. parsley, chopped
3 tbsp. minced olives
½ tsp. dill weed

Blend the cottage cheese and buttermilk in a blender, until smooth. Add the parsley, olives, tarragon and dill weed. Season to taste. Chill . . . and serve.

Silky's Nutty Fruit Cake

6 eggs, separated
1 tsp. vanilla
1 tsp. cinnamon
½ cup of small curd cottage
  cheese

⅓ cup of date powder or date
  sugar
pinch of cloves
1 tbsp. of carob powder

To use in the second step, also have ready . . .

½ cup of walnut chunks
½ cup of almonds, halved
½ cup of sunflower seeds
½ cup of sesame seeds

1 cup of raisins
¾ cup of dates, cut up
½ cup of figs, cut up
½ cup of prunes, cut up

First, beat the egg yolks well. Add the date sugar, a little at a time. Continue to beat. Add the vanilla, spices and cottage cheese. Beat well.

As the second step, mix the nuts, seeds and fruits into the yolk mixture. Fold in the six stiffly-beaten egg whites. Spread this entire mixture into a 7 x 16-inch Pyrex baking dish, which has been buttered. Place everything into a cold oven. Bake at 325 degrees, for 25 minutes. Test with a straw. Do not over-bake. Remove the fruit cake from the oven, and let it cool in the baking dish. This cake tastes best when it is eaten on the following day. Cut it into quarters, and wrap them in Saran wrap. Store in your refrigerator. Notice that this cake contains no flour, no sugar, no salt—no fat! And, it will keep fresh for weeks!

Carrot Yogurt Cake

2 cups of whole wheat pastry flour
½ cup of wheat germ
½ cup of bran
1 tsp. baking soda
2 tsp. cinnamon
¼ tsp. nutmeg
2 eggs, beaten

1 cup of grated carrots
1 cup of yogurt
½ cup of fresh orange juice
½ cup of molasses
½ cup of raisins
½ cup of sunflower seeds

Combine the ingredients, and beat well. Use an 8-inch square baking pan. Bake at 325 degrees, for one hour.

Fluffy Rice Pudding

½ cup of rice
(brown or white)
1 quart of milk
1 tbsp. of butter
2 tsp. of vanilla

2 eggs
½ cup of date sugar or raw sugar
¾ cup of raisins

Place milk, rice, and butter in the top of a double boiler. Cook for two hours, stirring frequently. Beat the eggs well. Beat the raw sugar, or date sugar, into the eggs. Combine hot mixture and eggs. Slowly pour the hot mixture into serving bowls or individual dishes. Sprinkle cinnamon on top. Decorate with colorful bits or slices of fresh fruit.

The tastes and eating habits of the American people have undergone some great changes in the past 35 years. Look at the popular fads which have swept the nation . . .

Fast food chains have promoted Mexican foods, now selling millions of tacos and enchiladas. The current rage is for croissants and quiche. Chinese restaurants have opened everywhere, tempting our palates with Cantonese, Mandarin and Szechuan cooking. And we've been invaded by the Japanese chefs, who bombard us with sushi, tempura, and raw fish delicacies.

Since we have acquired a liking for so many types of Oriental dishes, I decided to conclude this recipe section of my book by featuring . . .

ORIENTAL VEGETABLE DELIGHT
(A Crunchy Creation You Can Stir-Fry)

For this lively tasting treat, use these ingredients:

½ cup diced onion
½ cup sliced mushrooms
¼ cup diced green bell pepper
¼ cup diced red bell pepper
½ tsp. butter
½ cup Jicama or
    Jerusalem artichoke

1 cup sliced celery
1 cup sliced zucchini squash
1 cup shredded cabbage
¼ cup whole pea pods
¼ tbsp. natural soy sauce
½ cup whole almonds

Using a frying pan or wok, sauté the onion in butter. Add the mushrooms, and the red and green bell pepper. Sauté until lightly browned. Stir often. Add celery, zucchini, cabbage and pea pods. Keep at medium heat. Do not overcook. Lastly, add bean sprouts, Jicama or Jerusalem artichoke. Season with soy sauce, to taste.

Serve with cooked brown rice. Garnish with whole raw almonds. (This recipe can be changed, to substitute other vegetables which are in season.)

The beauty of this recipe—for cooking mixed vegetables, Oriental-style—is that you can do numerous variations of this dish. Take some thinly-sliced chicken breasts, sauté them in a bit of butter, and serve them on top of the vegetables as a garnish.

Or, broil some chicken legs and breasts, and arrange them around the vegetables, like a casserole.

Just be sure that the vegetables are undercooked, keep them crisp. Vary the mix . . . try yellow zucchini, green zucchini, crooked-neck squash or summer squash.

For another enjoyable version, you can sauté some scallops, shrimp, or crab in a little butter—to serve over the vegetables.

———————————

As I was writing the above recipe—with its Oriental overtones—I was reminded of a remarkable eating experience which I had in San Francisco. Let me recall for you . . .

THE INSPIRING STORY OF DR. DONG

I was the man who came to dinner. My host was an Oriental gentleman, who had invited me to his home. He was now in the kitchen, personally preparing some Chinese food, according to an ancient recipe.

His name was Dr. Collin Dong, and he lived in a large house on Telegraph Hill, furnished with many priceless antiques. And he had a jade collection of museum quality.

Dr. Dong was then, and is now, a very respected physician. He had graduated from Stanford University, never dreaming he would become a victim of arthritis.

For seven years, after medical school, Dr. Dong practiced medicine in San Francisco. Then, at the age of 35, he was suddenly stricken with both arthritis and dermatitis. He developed excruciating pain in his shoulders and other bodily joints.

One day, Dr. Dong looked in the mirror. He had lost most of his hair. The skin on his face was cracked, swollen, inflamed. For three years he tried every conceivable method of relief. Rheumatologists he consulted placed him on aspirin, analgesics, and every form of therapy. Nothing helped.

Finally, the Chinese doctor found the answer all by himself. He tells how he remembered a certain saying found in Chinese medical literature: "BING CHUNG HOW YUP, WOH CHUNG HOW CHUT."

Translated, that means: *"Sickness enters through the mouth, and catastrophe comes out of the mouth."*

DIET. Proper diet. Good nutrition seemed the logical way . . . so Dr. Dong changed his eating habits. He gave up processed foods, avoided those which had artificial flavoring, additives, preservatives.

Soon, Dr. Dong returned to good health. Today,

he is adamant about one fact: his recovery was *not* a case of temporary "spontaneous remission." His arthritis did not occur again. It is now 48 years later. Dr. Dong is 83 years old! Spry, happy, and still free of arthritic pain.

As I sat with Dr. Dong, for dinner, he told me that through the years he has treated thousands of cases of rheumatic diseases. He has told them the importance of nutrition, loud and clear.

Some years ago, Dr. Dong published his views and a collection of his recommended recipes. The volume—entitled: "The Arthritic's Cookbook"—is distributed in soft-cover by Bantam Books.

In the not too distant future, I plan to travel to the Orient. Research on arthritis is underway in Japan and China. I intend to examine the progress being made by their scientists. It's encouraging that everyone now realizes that arthritis is a worldwide problem.

I hope you remember what I've told you about Dr. Dong. Because he is unique.

His is a success story which can't be denied. This man is a doctor, *and* a former arthritic. He *knows* that proper nutrition accomplished a permanent solution for his rheumatic illness.

Just last week, I spoke with Dr. Dong again, by telephone. I hope that I am as healthy as he is, when I reach age 83.

FOR SPECIAL SUGGESTIONS REGARDING THE MENUS AND RECIPES IN THIS CHAPTER, SEE PAGE 180.
You'll find additional facts—helpful hints on how to cook and prepare meals properly—by turning to Chapter XVI, Pages 180 to 185.

NOT AS BENEFICIAL. WHY? SEE page 145

SUGGESTED TO RELIEVE CONSTIPATION

IS A NEW HEALTH DRINK

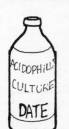

To make it,
you add acidophilus.
SEE PAGE 148.

DATE ON BOTTLE
IS IMPORTANT

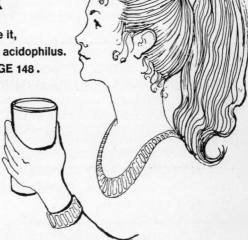

ANOTHER WAY TO KEEP REGULAR, TRY SOME FRESH FRUIT AND BERRIES COMBINED WITH PLAIN YOGURT.

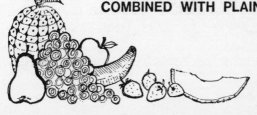

143

CHAPTER XII

Better Health . . . By The Process of Elimination

Your physical fitness—your ability to enjoy life, from day to day—depends largely on whether or not your body can eliminate wastes in a normal manner.

We all suffer, occasionally, from constipation. Arthritics are particularly prone to this malady . . . they often report that their intestines and bowels do not function with *regularity.*

That's the key word. Regularity. How can we achieve a "regular" schedule and avoid constipation?

I will make some suggestions in this chapter. My research on how to combat constipation has continued for 30 years. In my first book, I devoted 20 pages to this topic—because it is such a major problem for people who have arthritis.

Noted rheumatologists conducted experiments among their arthritic patients to determine whether faulty diet is the cause of chronic constipation. Doctor Ralph Pemberton (see pages 18 and 19 of this book) restricted "inferior-type" starches—like candy and cake from the diets of his patients. Their bowel movements improved.

Dr. A. A. Fletcher of Toronto, Canada, reported

144

his findings in *The Journal of Laboratory and Clinical Medicine.* He recommended Vitamin B as beneficial.

According to Dr. Fletcher, constipation can be caused by vitamin deficiencies. You need Vitamin B, specifically, or else your bowel may break down and have less digestive power.

Wherever I travel these days, lecturing, victims of arthritis volunteer the information that they have frequent attacks of constipation. To alleviate this condition, many people are trying yogurt in their daily diet. Repeatedly, they ask me for my honest opinion about yogurt. So, here are the facts . . .

THE HISTORY OF YOGURT. CAN IT EASE CONSTIPATION?

Fermented milk products, including yogurt, have been a boon to health for hundreds of years. In many nations—India, Turkey, Iran, etc.—this food has been popular for generations.

It is true that yogurt has antibiotic properties which tend to restore normal intestinal equilibrium. As insurance against digestive upsets, I do recommend *whole milk yogurt.*

Unfortunately, several new types of yogurt have been manufactured and are now being heavily adver-tisted on television. These new "variations" of the product may taste more "custardy"—but they have lost much of their effectiveness as a laxative.

Non-fat yogurt has been over-processed, in my opinion, and it can cause flatulence. Fruit syrups have been whipped into some brands of yogurt (with preservatives to prolong shelf-life, no doubt.) I do encourage you to eat *plain, natural yogurt*. You can embellish the taste yourself, by adding sliced fruit.

Many doctors now acklowledge the health-giving qualities of yogurt. They began to react favorably toward this food after they studied the research work performed by one man. Let's give credit where credit is due. The acceptance of yogurt was achieved by a Russian.

Elie Metchnikoff is the respected bacteriologist who discovered the benefits of yogurt. Metchnikoff shared a Nobel prize in 1908. His studies proved the effect of lactic acid bacteria within the digestive tract. He concluded that yogurt arrests intestinal putrefaction. Now, the medical world agrees.

Commercial manufacturers, in the United States, create yogurt from fresh, homogenized, pasteurized cow's milk. They add two types of bacteria to the milk, causing it to ferment. By adding *Lactobacillus bulgaricus* and *Streptococcus lactis,* a culturing process takes place in temperature-controlled incubators.

The bacteria multiply, lactic acid causes the fluid milk to thicken, and the result is yogurt.

If you are trying to lose weight, it's helpful, because unflavored yogurt contains only a few calories per serving.

While I favor yogurt, I continue to oppose any diet which permits too much refined sugar. During a recent lecture, I told how sugar disrupts the microorganisms of the intestinal flora—which are trying to break down your food as part of the digestive process. If you block that process, you will surely experience constipation.

After that lecture, came a pleasant surprise . . .

As I prepared to leave the lecture hall, a woman walked up to me and introduced herself. She had been listening, in the audience. That day, she had traveled a considerable distance to attend the event.

"I want to thank you," she said. "Your previous book did a great service for my mother. Here is a letter I wrote . . . to express my deep appreciation."

The letter reads:

"My mother went to a medical doctor in great pain. He diagnosed osteoarthritis and X-rays showed spurs on her spine.

"He gave her a prescription, but being a Carlton Frederick's fan, she was very bothered by taking drugs. So, as a last resort, she decided to go to the library, to see if she could find some helpful information, and found 'Arthritis and Common Sense.'

"Mom is the kind of person who has great self-discipline, and when Dale Alexander said 'no sugar' that meant *no* sugar—even on Christmas Day. She followed this regime faithfully until all the pain was gone, and has continued with the cod liver oil.

"A few years later she went to see a nephew who is a doctor, and he took X-rays and found no spurs, and told her she had a 'photographic spine.'

"Mom was born in 1899 and has a degree in Home Economics from Cornell University. Back in the

1920's, when she taught in public schools, she always put nutrition into her classes—not to the delight of her students who wanted to get on to making goodies and eating them.''

Mrs. C.K.
La Mirada, California

It is moments like these—comments from grateful readers—that brighten my life, year after year. If my work is achieving results for *people,* then I shall continue to share my knowledge with renewed spirit.

In an effort to help constipated arthritics I have carefully designed a special formula. Printed below is a mixture of ingredients, which you can prepare in a blender, to stimulate greater regularity.

Formula To Combat Constipation

½ cup to one full cup of Whole Milk
1 raw egg
2 tbsp. Liquid Acidophilus Culture
2 tbsp. Bran (heaping) (Fibre for Bulk)
1 tbsp. Raw Wheat Germ (heaping) (For Fibre & Vitamin B)
1 tsp. Brewer's Yeast (level) (For Vitamin B complex)
¼ Ripe Papaya (Papain) (For Digestive Aid)
1 tbsp. Psyllium Husks (Fibre) (To soften stool)
1 Ripe Banana (whole banana, if small, or ½ large banana)
(The above amounts, prepared in a blender, serve one person.)

Additional Suggestions

When you feel you need it, substitute this formula drink in place of your regular breakfast. Or, take it each night just before you retire. Continue drinking it, once a day, until your regularity returns.

In place of papaya plus banana, you may use six large, raw pitted prunes . . . or six large Mission figs.

To enhance peristalsis, add 1 to 2 tablespoons of plain yogurt. Do not use non-fat, low-fat or flavored yogurts. You may add 1 tablespoon of raw honey for sweetening.

Brewer's yeast and raw wheat germ, to newcomers, present a new taste factor. If you wish, you can begin using it in smaller quantities.

You are trying to speed up the transit time of your food as it passes through your gastro-intestinal tract. Use at least 2 tablespoonsful of Acidophilus Culture.

READ THE LABEL. Be sure to select a natural acidophilus culture (containing Lactobacillus Caucasicus and Lactobacillus Bulgaricus) in milk whey. High grade acidophilus is alive with millions of hardy, viable (live) organisms.

This product should first be placed in a blender. It is not as effective if mixed in water, fruit juice or vegetable juice. And it will not be as helpful if you take the acidophilus directly from a spoon, after a meal.

Check the date on the label. The live organisms have a limited life span. After about six months "on the shelf" the value of the product may be diminished.

The Vitamin B (in wheat germ) will gradually assist in correcting bowel-muscle tone. Bran helps to make bulky stools. Remember, you are seeking to achieve a certain *type* of stool, not copious amounts. For most people, one bowel movement per day is normal. However, missing a day should not cause great alarm.

Stool quantity may be less on a fish-type diet. Your bowel movement should be nearly odorless. Try to establish an approximate set-time each day, for this natural function.

I firmly believe that *both arthritis and constipation can be caused by the same dietary mistakes!*

CHAPTER XIII

Chiropractors . . . Take A Closer Look

"The pain is worse in my joints, and my back hurts! Should I go see a chiropractor?"

Perhaps you have asked yourself that question a dozen times. But you have always hesitated, just a little afraid to seek chiropractic help. The idea of someone "manipulating" your spine and joints may seem like "a last resort" . . . a desperate form of therapy.

I'd like to correct that impression, and suggest that victims of arthritis can sometimes benefit by consulting a chiropractor. The men and women who have graduated from chiropractic colleges are members of a proud profession. Most of them have had 4,480 classroom hours—studying psychology, chemistry, anatomy, pathology, bacteriology and similar subjects. They have *earned* their degrees as "Doctors of Chiropractic."

More than 70,000,000 chiropractic treatments are given every year! This method to restore good health has become the second largest healing art in the world.

You can feel secure, because chiropractors are licensed by law in all 50 states and Canada. Most states also require them to take postgraduate courses before renewing their licenses.

In this chapter, let me show how the work of chiropractors can be effective against arthritis.

To acquire accurate information for this book— to study the latest chiropractic techniques being used on patients—I wanted to watch one particular doctor at work. He is considered one of the nation's foremost authorities on this science of healing.

So, let's meet the man, in person. He is Dr. John F. Thie . . . and we shall now visit his chiropractic institution, located in Pasadena, California.

As I drive my car through downtown Pasadena, the place seems familiar. You would recognize the landmarks, because they are shown on television each New Year's Day. These streets are the site of "The Tournament of Roses" Parade, a spectacular TV event.

Doctor Thie has built an organization which includes 15 chiropractors and technicians. They have treated thousands of patients in Pasadena, and the Thie method of "Touch for Health" is published in a manual that is now being followed throughout the world.

Before we meet with Doctor Thie in his office, let me give you some background facts about this form of therapy.

The term "chiropractic" is based on two Greek words—"cheir" and "praktikas"—which mean "done by hand." Careful manipulation of the spine and other bodily joints is how chiropractors achieve results.

For a more complete definition, let me quote the American Chiropractic Association. They describe this science as one "which utilizes the inherent recuperative powers of the body, and the relationship between the musculoskeletal structures and functions of the body, particularly of the spinal column and the nervous system, in the restoration and maintenance of health."

In plain English, people should realize that a connection exists between their spine and their internal organs. Fix one, you help the other.

Remember, however, that chiropractors do *not* treat diseases. They help a patient's body to heal itself. Their goal is to assist your body, make it gain a higher level of function and resistance to diseases.

For arthritics, this would be an achievement in itself. To have more movement in their joints, and reduced pain.

If you still have some doubts, and you tend to shy away from chiropractors, here's one key fact you might consider . . . Some very intelligent people have included regular chiropractic care as part of their lives. Among the famous patients—who trusted this form of treatment—were Thomas Edison, Herbert Hoover, Harry S Truman, John D. Rockefeller, Sr., Reverend Norman Vincent Peale, Mahatma Gandhi and Ronald Reagan.

Eleanor Roosevelt used to visit a chiropractor once a month. Also recognizing the advantages of this science are ladies like Lucille Ball, Julie Andrews, Marlo Thomas, and scores of prominent entertainers.

All these thoughts were going through my mind, as I parked my car, and walked into the office building which houses the Thie Chiropractic Corporation.

Join me, as we tour this facility. We shall meet Dr. Thie and his associates. The staff includes eight other doctors, a nurse, three physical therapists, and five chiropractic assistants.

Dr. Thie welcomes us, personally. As we sit in his modern office, he gives us a statement which clearly defines his entire field of work:

"Chiropractors do not approach the health of the person in the same manner as the medical profession. They are looking at the same thing through different eyes.

"Medical science takes a dead body and looks at the processes that it went through to cause it to die. They look for, find, and name a disease, and then work backwards to try to cure it.

"The chiropractor works from the opposite premise, that of normalcy. He says, 'Here is what a normal person looks like. Let's try to put you back into the normal position.' "

THE TWO REQUISITES . . . EDUCATION AND MODERN EQUIPMENT

Can a Chiropractor help a victim of arthritis? Can he ease "the pains you have learned to live with?"

According to Dr. Thie, the answer is "Yes!" But the chiropractic doctor must be highly trained, at a recognized college. And he also needs the proper tools—including scientific X-Ray machinery.

"Postural X-Ray will reveal past injuries—the traumatic events and stresses that began the arthritic or other degenerative processes.

"Without the postural X-Ray examination, easily correctable problems can be missed—and otherwise excellent nutritional approaches take much longer to get results."

On another floor, in Dr. Thie's building, is an elaborate X-Ray room. After a patient is examined and X-rayed, trained technicians place the "pictures" in an automatic developer. Five minutes later, the doctor is able to "read" the X-rays and interpret them.

Dr. Thie takes us into each department, to view the equipment. Therapy available includes diathermy, ultrasound, sine wave galvanism, cervical and lumbar spinal traction and hydroculators.

With this modern technology, Dr. Thie and his colleagues can treat hundreds of patients each week.

In the X-Ray examination room, Dr. Thie again emphasizes what can be accomplished. He reveals this new technique:

"The 14 x 36-inch standing X-Ray studies both front to back and lateral—giving more information about the posture of an arthritic sufferer than any other single X-Ray study. It allows the patient to be seen in standing balance.

"With this study, special exercises can be prescribed specifically for the patient's underlying problems. The degenerative changes of the spine can be visualized as a whole.

"Often times, lifts can be added inside the shoes—or having one heel shortened—to allow walking to treat the patient and relax tightened muscles.

"We often employ chiropractic manipulation— and specific muscle balancing by Touch for Health Applied Kinesiology—and restore motion and strength to muscles very rapidly. Then, with proper nutritional support, the person can be relieved of their arthritis."

Dr. Thie is firmly convinced that his patients must have *proper nutritional support* . . . this is a prime requirement for any patient trying to conquer pain.

When a person seeks treatment from Dr. Thie, the patient is often asked to undergo a dietary survey and mineral analysis. You are given a specific form, on which you list everything you eat during a one-week period. This list is then placed into a computer, and is analyzed for what nutrients are in the food.

A hair sample is then taken—to see if those nutrients have been properly absorbed, digested, and transported to the cells.

Dr. Thie and his group of chiropractors recently issued a Bulletin to each of their patients. It read:

"Lately there has been a lot of commotion about good nutrition—vitamins, proteins and health foods.

Much new information is coming out all the time, but the basics are clear . . .

"Proper nutrition is absolutely essential to good health. The simplest guide is *eat only whole foods.* If a food is processed or broken down into another form—avoid it. Stay as close to the natural state of the food as is reasonable.

"The ground rule is always, *fresh food is best.* Frozen food is usually better than canned, but the goal is to eat a variety of natural foods in their natural state and to eat all the different parts of them."

————————

The above credo is totally correct. I extend my congratulations to Dr. Thie. He arrived at these conclusions years ago, independent of my work.

During our meeting at his office, Dr. Thie and I discussed many dietary factors . . . ideas which could affect all arthritics.

Here are some special comments made by Dr. Thie:

"Regarding artificial sweeteners, I feel that they should not be recommended. The chewing of foods for longer periods of time will satisfy the sweet taste—by allowing the enzyme ptyalin (in the mouth) to convert the starch in most foods into sugar. The sweetness will be tasted.

"Fresh fruits can also be utilized for that sweet satisfaction. I agree with you, completely, on not recommending juices. I believe that the complex carbohydrates in the whole fruits are much better, rather than the refined carbohydrate of the juices."

Next, our conversation turned to the topic of *iodine*. Dr. Thie made his views quite clear. He said:

"I believe that there is a widespread deficiency of iodine in the world today. Iodine is lost—even when it is present in foods in its free form—by the process of the foods and especially the cooking.

"Iodine goes into a vapor at 186 degrees F. Thus, the electrical balance of the cells is lost. The halogens, which maintain this balance, are upset by the lack of iodine.

"When the electrical balance is upset, cellular malnutrition begins. Foods cannot be adequately absorbed at the cellular level. Tissue rebuilding is impaired and scar tissues are substituted. Due to lack of iodine, oxidation does not take place sufficiently. Then, toxic wastes are accumulated.

"Toxic wastes create a greater burden on the lymphatic and hepatic systems. This toxicity causes a reduction of energy, and fatigue."

Perhaps you will heed this warning—and the other suggestions made by Dr. Thie—based on his 27 years of experience as an expert chiropractor. He is a graduate of USC, and he has served as President of the Los Angeles County Chiropractic Society.

It is evident that many of his findings have run parallel to mine—dietary discoveries made during the past three decades.

Nutrition has become a major subject, now being taught at chiropractic colleges from coast to coast. I have already lectured at many of these institutions . . . at the National College of Chiropractic in Lombard, Illinois . . . at the Texas School of Chiropractic . . . at Logan Chiropractic College in Springfield, Missouri.

The message is finally sinking in: Patients *are* what they eat. Doctors should *study* this precept.

THE WAY TO GO . . . COLLEGE-TRAINED NUTRITIONISTS

There is one route we can follow, one road which could lead to better health for millions of Americans. We can start, now, by teaching nutrition at our largest colleges and universities. Let us graduate some well-trained experts who can prescribe proper diet to prevent illness.

Medical schools teach pharmacology—how to administer aspirin and pills. We need more college courses on how to select and eat nutritious foods.

This knowledge—about natural foods and intelligent dietary procedures—can even be taught by mail.

Correspondence courses are now being offered, and that's a good start in the right direction.

The best-known example of such an educational program is a series of courses now being circulated by the Donsbach University, School of Nutrition. More than 4,000 students, worldwide, have already had career training via this institution, which is located in Huntington Beach, California.

It is interesting to note that the University was founded by a chiropractor. Nearly 30 years ago, Dr. Kurt Donsbach was a student at Western States College of Chiropractic in Portland, Oregon. After graduation, he achieved a national reputation in that science. Through the years, he became convinced that better nutrition was the answer to many critical ailments.

Doctor Donsbach spoke out strongly in behalf of new approaches to solve medical problems. He earned the respect of his colleagues, and was elected as the Chairman of the Board of the National Health Federation. (See page 106.) He currently serves on the Board of Directors of NHF.

While gathering pertinent facts to include in this book, I met with Dr. Donsbach in his office at the University. He told me how the School of Nutrition has grown rapidly, since it was established back in 1977. The present enrollment includes students from Australia, South Africa, Japan, Saudi Arabia, Yugoslavia, and many other nations.

Serious interest in nutrition is expanding every year, circling the globe. Perhaps the day of awakening has arrived. I'm encouraged.

I hope these past few pages have enlightened some of my readers . . . causing you to have new respect for the highly-educated men and women who have become chiropractors.

You'll be seeing more Doctors of Chiropractic in the years ahead. In the United States there are now 17 colleges teaching this profession, with a total enrollment of nearly 11,000 students. I talked with the national headquarters of the American Chiropractic Association recently. Dr. Thomas Speer, their Director of Professional Services, told me that these colleges will graduate 2,400 chiropractors each year.

I can imagine the happy esteem that those 2,400 students will bring to their families. Their parents will share a special pride . . . because their sons and daughters decided to follow a career in the science of healing, serving their fellow human beings.

My own son made such a decision, and it was one of the most joyous moments of my life. He set out to become a psychologist. After graduating from Brown University in Rhode Island, he earned his Ph.D. degree at Claremont College in California. His chosen field is to work with children—victims of mental retardation and autism. Now, Dr. Dean Alexander is on the staff of a large hospital in California.

Yes, our hope for the future is with the young doctors of today. To achieve good health for all, we must build and expand our educational institutions. Support the college of your choice.

CHAPTER XIV

Experiments on Animals . . . To Solve Arthritis?

I love animals. The joy of raising a dog, or any house pet, begins in childhood. Having a lovable and faithful companion, like a dog or a cat, makes life more bearable for many senior citizens.

So, I soundly condemn any person who is guilty of cruelty to any creatures of God. I do not condone the slaughter of animals in the name of science. Some of the laboratory experiments now being performed on helpless animals are extremely savage and blood-thirsty. They are inflicting needless pain . . . the tests are too severe and too prolonged.

While I certainly sympathize with the goals of the ASPCA, and other groups which try to protect our animal population, I must also add that I do not propose that all animal experimentation should be prohibited. Many humans are alive today only because of medical research which utilized test animals. Discoveries have been made, to improve the health of mankind, at the cost of animal life.

Changing the eating habits of mice or rats can be done humanely. But don't implant a balloon catheter in the pulmonary artery of a conscious, non-sedated dog. All arthritis victims should be *thankful* to the animal world. There are many reasons why. For an authentic report, see the next page . . .

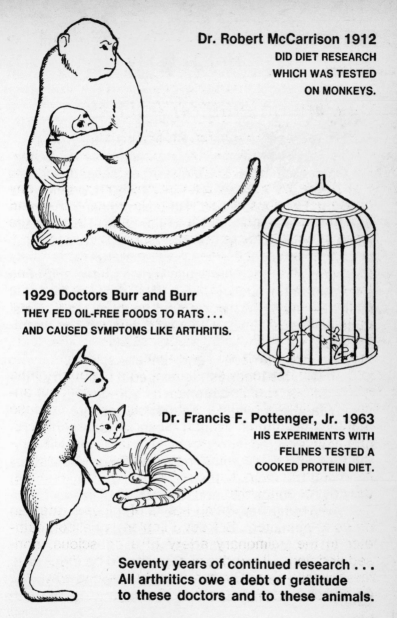

Dr. Robert McCarrison 1912
DID DIET RESEARCH
WHICH WAS TESTED
ON MONKEYS.

1929 Doctors Burr and Burr
THEY FED OIL-FREE FOODS TO RATS . . .
AND CAUSED SYMPTOMS LIKE ARTHRITIS.

Dr. Francis F. Pottenger, Jr. 1963
HIS EXPERIMENTS WITH
FELINES TESTED A
COOKED PROTEIN DIET.

Seventy years of continued research . . .
All arthritics owe a debt of gratitude
to these doctors and to these animals.

My main discussion of experiments performed on animals should certainly begin with the true story of *Dr. Robert McCarrison.*

He was British, and for his accomplishments he was knighted and became Sir Robert McCarrison.

For part of his career, he served as a Lieutenant Colonel in India. Dr. McCarrison carried out field and laboratory research in Kasauli during the years of 1912 and 1913. He was studying the relation between goiter, diet and infection. He later became fascinated with the diet of the Sikh people in India.

Why did these particular Indians have such fine physiques and such powers of endurance? Was it their diet? They ate wholemeal flour, milk products, fruits and vegetables, with a little meat on festive occasions.

Dr. McCarrison, and other scientists who agreed with his theories, developed a plan to try "the Sikh diet" on rats and monkeys.

Years ago, when I was doing research on the problem of arthritis, I found these facts in an old report. It was buried in the archives of a medical library. But I tracked down some more history on Dr. McCarrison and the monkey tests.

Two groups of monkeys were utilized. Those that were fed the Sikh diet remained healthy. But one group of ten monkeys had only autoclaved rice.

When food is "autoclaved" it is placed in an oven-like apparatus. Tremendous heat is turned on, under high pressure. This "overcooks" the food—the beneficial enzymes are deliberately destroyed.

The poor monkeys being fed autoclaved rice soon became ill.

Their meals were deficient in suitable protein, and lacked fat. Their "menu" was also excessively rich in starch. What happened was disastrous. All ten monkeys died.

For decades medical science has been warning us to pay attention to the oils in our daily diet. As far back as 1929 there was experimental research underway. *Dr. G.O. Burr* and *Dr. M.M. Burr* were proving that an oil-free diet is dangerous.

They decided to use rats as their test animals. By feeding the rats on oil-free foods for 70 to 90 days, the sad creatures became victims of a dozen ailments. Kidney damage was evident. Dry and scaly skin became an early symptom. The rats then began to suffer from swollen and inflamed joints.

The same afflictions which now strike arthritic humans were being duplicated in laboratory animals! The rats did receive adequate amounts of protein, carbohydrates, minerals, etc.——so the only thing missing from their food was *the essential oils.*

These findings——which should have alerted the entire medical profession——were published in the *Journal of Biological Chemistry.*

But more than 30 years passed by, before the next key development.

It was 1963 when *Dr. Francis F. Pottenger, Jr.,* conducted a significant set of experiments. He did his work with cats. The results were highly critical of "cooked" protein and the way it destroys an otherwise healthful diet.

Dr. Pottenger fed groups of cats in two separate ways. Some were given a raw protein diet, while others received cooked animal protein. His observations, on 109 cats, continued for five years. All of the felines that were placed on cooked protein soon had diseases which were similar to those seen in man.

The unfortunate animals developed progressive liver impairment, arthritis, loss of hair and teeth—plus the first generation of kittens were abnormal. By the second generation, many in the litter were born dead. The mother cats then became sterile, so there was no third generation.

Simultaneously, other groups of cats were fed on raw protein foods ... and they went purring along in very good health.

The parallels to what I've been saying in this book are obvious. Don't overcook, eat more raw foods.

THE OTHER SIDE OF THE COIN ... ABUSED ANIMALS!

We must admit that many laboratories can be accused of using excessive torture in the way they conduct animal tests.

There is no excuse for brutality, nor for seizing unclaimed pet animals from an animal shelter to sacrifice in deadly experiments.

I cringe when I hear how someone's pet dog has had bacteria injected into its brain, until abscesses result. As the abscesses grow, their development is monitored by sophisticated X-ray techniques.

Cats are implanted with brain electrodes, their windpipes are connected to the outside via a hole in the neck. Various drugs are then injected, causing the cat to have breathing abnormalities, so a lab worker can study the effects.

One last example . . . We've all heard about the cosmetics company which placed substances into the eyes of rabbits. While the heads of the bunnies were held in stocks to restrict their movement, chemicals were dropped into their eyes—causing ulcerations and even blindness.

Few people realize that there has been a vast increase in animal testing. It's happening, now, across America. Currently, an estimated *four billion dollars* in Federal tax money is spent each year on animal experimentation.

The Congress of the United States is beginning to ask questions. The House of Representatives Sub-Committee on Science and Technology conducted extensive hearings on the topic of animal research. Here are some excerpts from the actual testimony . . . these are statements by Congressmen:

"Sixty-five million animals die in the name of scientific research annually in the United States. This is a slaughter of incredible dimensions. Tens of millions of those animals suffer intense and prolonged agony while being subjected to unnecessary or duplicative experimentation." *Hon. Brian Donnelly of Massachusetts.*

"We do not need to spend research money to

find out what we already know, nor do we need to spend money for poorly designed research that will not tell us what we do need to know. . . . The issue, Mr. Chairman, is not scientific freedom but scientific accountability." *Hon. Tom Lantos of California.*

"Many of these animals suffer needless cruelty and suffering in laboratories because researchers are often not aware of, or do not have access to, alternative methods. . . . Moreover, many animals are senselessly subjected to protracted pain during duplicative and unnecessary experiments." *Hon. Ted Weiss of New York.*

Of all the testimony given, I liked the biting comment made by *Representative G. William Whitehurst of Virginia.* He said: "It is clear that additional safeguards are necessary to insure the continued humane treatment of animals and to end practices of abuse. . . . For in medical research, it is not always easy to determine at the edge of a scalpel which is the 'dumb animal.' "

REVISE THE ANIMAL TESTS . . . OR END THEM!

For all arthritics, everywhere, I now lodge a protest. The present methods of animal experimentation are wasteful and improperly conducted. Laboratories have been feeding their test subjects the *wrong* liquids and *incorrect* diets. Scientists, a vast majority of them, have made detailed dietary observations based on a faulty premise. They have ignored oil-bearing foods. No wonder the animals develop "arthritis" and suffer.

For 30 years, the laboratory technicians have given animals water-based and milk-based diets. Just hoping to learn the nutritional effects. Why don't they feed the creatures some carbonated beverages and chart the damage done? *Prove* the dangers that soda pop and overcooked foods can cause to muscles, joints, and digestive organs. Then, *warn* the public what to avoid!

Perhaps, throughout this Chapter, I have sounded ambivalent—half for and half against animal experiments. In a way, I do have mixed emotions on this subject. I have shown you how beneficial lessons can be learned through the use of monkeys, mice and cats. Doctors McCarrison, Burr and Pottenger were on the right track. That was years ago. *When are modern medical men going to follow up on those experiments?*

Dietary research can be done with animals. On a limited basis, humanely.

I hope my readers will join me in a campaign to urge better laws for the protection of animals. There are many organizations working toward this goal. The Humane Society of the United States now has more than 200,000 members. The National Anti-Vivisection Society has a membership of nearly 50,000 concerned Americans.

Another dedicated group is The Fund for Animals, Inc. Some of the facts and "quotes" in this Chapter were originally assembled by their Science Advisor, Dr. Michael Giannelli. He issued an effective report—against the use of laboratory animals—deploring many experiments being done at the University of California.

The public *cares*. For example, four years ago, a new group was formed, with just 18 members. They called themselves *People for Ethical Treatment of Animals*. Today, they have 23,000 supporters!

To reinforce our love for animals, we need to remember just one fact: "Pain is pain, whether it is inflicted on man or beast."

CHAPTER XV

Your Questions . . . My Answers. A Dialogue Between Us

By now, you have read more than 150 pages of this book. So, you have probably formed your own opinion about my credibility. You may have decided that my dietary plan sounds very plausible, but you are still wondering whether or not you should try this nutritional approach.

Perhaps you have some *specific questions.* You are certainly entitled to seek answers about the type of arthritis that affects you most. I welcome your inquiries, by mail and by phone.

I receive hundreds of letters. Later, in this Chapter, I'll let you "read my mail" . . . and some of the matters discussed may be the very same topics that are on your mind.

I always accept any invitation from a television commentator—or from the host of a radio "talk show"—because such interviews often give me a chance to speak directly with actual victims of arthritis. Many of the programs will announce a telephone number, so that listeners can call in. That's a great way for you to have a chat with Dale Alexander.

For instance, I recently took part in such a broadcast on Radio Station WGBS in Miami. From a

tape recording which was made, here are some highlights . . .

(On this particular program, the Host conducting
the interview was Barry Young. He has a huge audience, thousands of listeners throughout southern
Florida. One of the first phone calls came from a lady
named Mirta. She had one main worry . . . and her
question is one that I hear frequently.)

MIRTA: Does cod liver oil make you fat?

DALE: Any oil—whether it's cod liver oil, soybean oil,
safflower or sunflower oil—has calories. But by
taking cod liver oil my way, you are emulsifying it
first. Do not, I repeat, do not take it from the spoon.
(Emulsifying the oil) will take it around the liver—so
that it does not act as a calorie. If it goes around the
liver, it oils the skin, the joints, the hair, the eyes,
makes new ear wax . . . it creates lubrication and
healing power. Only if you have the correct diet
which goes with the cod liver oil. It does not have
anything to do with putting on weight.

MIRTA: Another question. I have colitis. If I take cod
liver oil, will that make it worse?

DALE: Once you have colitis, you must mix the cod
liver oil with milk, not with orange juice. Use two tablespoonsful of whole milk. Get yourself a little
baby jar, put in two tablespoons of the milk, and
then one tablespoon of the cod liver oil . . . and
shake it into a froth. And take it thirty minutes before breakfast.

BARRY YOUNG: I want you to remember, everyone listening to the show today, that Dale is not going to prescribe anything for you. He's not going to play doctor with you. He's going to answer in generalities . . . He can give you some basic information about what has worked for other people. But, if you are taking medication, don't begin or end any kind of medication without talking to your medical doctor first. And I'm sure Dale will agree with that all the way.

DALE: Exactly!

(The next telephone call—which I answered, on the air—was from a lady who spoke with a British accent. Her name was Valerie, and she now lives in the Miami area.)

VALERIE: In England, during the last war, all the adults were on rations. But the babies were given, by the Government, free rations of cod liver oil and orange juice. So, they were really ahead, weren't they?
DALE: Yes, that's very true.
VALERIE: Incidentally, I drink loads of milk. I've got a gorgeous skin—not my opinion, other people's. I also have some marvelous grapefruit, which I do eat. And I'm wondering if I can substitute fresh grapefruit juice, suitably strained, with the cod liver oil?
DALE: No. You cannot mix the cod liver oil with grapefruit juice. It's ten times more caustic than orange juice.

VALERIE: I was taking 50,000 milligrams of Vitamin A in capsule form. That's no good, eh?

DALE: You can use the capsules as an adjunct—as part of the energy process of your body. Capsules are surrounded by a gelatin material. It's digested and sent to the liver. It has very little to do with the oiling of your eyes or skin.

(This transcript of the Miami radio broadcast is just a brief sample of what was said on the air. The telephones kept ringing constantly, and I talked with listeners for two solid hours.)

Your telephone calls continue to impress me. Your inquiries are often very incisive, probing . . . you demand common sense answers.

It is quite possible that you and I may meet someday, at one of my lectures. During my personal appearance tours, I welcome the chance to converse "one-on-one" with any person who has arthritis.

Watch your local newspapers, in the months ahead, and you may find news stories which announce that I will be lecturing in your town or city.

At the end of each of my lectures, I try to set aside time to accept questions from the audience. I have held open discussions, in public, on almost every type of arthritic ailment known to man. I have learned from the questions asked . . . and I hope my audiences have benefited from the advice I gave them regarding their nutritional needs.

By far the best way to contact me is by mail. Between trips, when I return from lecture events, I try to answer your letters individually. I invite you to write to me, personally——in care of my Publisher, whose address appears on the last page of this book.

———————————

Recently, my friendly mailman brought me dozens of letters. Let's "open" a few of them . . . and read them, together. What questions will these arthritics ask? Here's a typical letter . . . from a lady in Texas . . .

Q. The four-hour waiting period (for drinking water after meals) is quite long. What can I drink to quench my thirst? I live in hot, humid Houston.

A. Even during hot and sticky weather, I'm afraid my rules must still apply. But try drinking more water upon arising——ten minutes *before* breakfast. When thirsty, you may enjoy chewing some wet celery, or an apple.

Another suggestion is to drink a vegetable juice. Like carrot juice. Or, mix buttermilk with freshly-squeezed orange juice——with the pulp still in the juice. Liquids like these, with low surface tension, can be assimilated more easily——without fighting the dietary oils which your food provides.

The next letter asks a question which concerns many people:

Q. Will taking cod liver oil raise my cholesterol level any higher than it already is?

A. Cod liver oil has no cholesterol. A normal person has a blood serum cholesterol level of 150 to 250 milligrams per 100 centimeters of blood. If you take cod liver oil properly and observe a correct diet, your cholesterol level will actually go *down* within a few months.

A letter-writer, who may be Italian, asked this next question . . .

Q. You never mention such foods as Pasta, Spaghetti, Macaroni, or Pizza. Can they be eaten, in moderation?

A. Of course. But it is best if they are of the whole grain variety.

Q. The only thing, Mr. Alexander, is that for years I've had this dry mouth. I can't swallow food unless I wash it down with a liquid——which is coffee, milk, or water. I drink no tea or carbonated beverages.

A. A suggestion: drink herbal tea. Perhaps one or two cups, five to ten minutes before every meal. Do this for 10 days or so, and it should help.

I also recommend that you see your doctor. Have him check to determine whether you have Sjogren's syndrome. This "dry mouth" ailment (Sjogren's syndrome) is a form of rheumatoid

PUBLISHER'S NOTE: The excerpts from the Miami radio broadcast, quoted in this chapter, accurately reflect the topics discussed. The questions and answers were edited slightly, primarily to meet the limited space requirements of this book manuscript. Minor editing also took place on the letters which readers wrote to the author—so that each question is stated concisely.

arthritis, occurring chiefly in post-menopausal women.

Q. What about canned soups, to which water has been added? Should they be included in the diet?

A. Yes. Soup is generally consumed when it's warm, at the beginning of the meal. Soup is considered to be a "low" surface-tension liquid . . . and that's compatible with my dietary plan.

Q. Can I have sweets twice a week?

A. Providing your arthritis is not of the rheumatoid type. It would be advisable that you try "natural" sweets. Like sugarless, flourless cake . . . see the recipe on page 136 of this book. Another route is to enjoy melon, in season.

Q. I have bursitis in both shoulders. What brought this condition on?

A. You may have imbalanced the amounts of calcium and phosphorus in your body. This could happen by eating an over-abundance of sweets. When a blood sample is taken from a healthy person, and sent to a laboratory, it will show 10 parts of calcium to 4 parts of phosphorus. Too many sweets in your diet can knock this 10-to-4 ratio out of kilter.

Another possible cause could be that you lack sufficient Vitamin D oils in your bloodstream.

Q. Are the following foods allowed on your diet? Peaches? Rice? Apricot juice?

A. Fresh peaches are fine. Yes, to rice and whole grains. Enjoy apricot juice, occasionally.

Q. I am 78, and I'm a recent widow. I have sciatica rheumatism. Can I be helped by your program?

A. I certainly believe that correct nutrition can have a favorable effect. Why? Because the sciatic nerve—the largest nerve in our bodies—is covered and insulated by myelin. This is a fatty substance, which can benefit from proper foods and eating habits. Also, you should be particularly careful to avoid drinking tannic-acid teas and carbonated beverages.

Q. Is natural, freshly-made peanut butter—made on the premises, in health food stores—acceptable?

A. Yes. Once or twice a week, that's one of my favorite snacks. Instead of bread, try spreading the peanut butter on whole grain crackers. Very tasty.

Q. In the hospital, they keep giving me juices. Why are you against juices?

A. I am *not* against reasonable quantities of *vegetable* juices. But I fully condemn frozen, canned, or concentrated citric juices.

Q. I have never had any problem with my throat. But, I now talk a "little hoarse." Will the oil help?

A. For your throat condition try an emulsion of cod liver oil—rather than pure cod liver oil. Take it every night, by the tablespoonful. Do not swallow it. Let it stick to the roof of your mouth—to lubricate and heal, while you sleep. See page 264.

Go to a throat specialist, to make sure that dryness is the only problem. Seek medical help, if you have any persistent cough.

Q. I'm afraid to continue cod liver oil until I know if it is a saturated or unsaturated fat.

A. Cod liver oil is a polyunsaturated marine oil. You should avoid oils that turn "hard" at room temperature. Such oils (found in margarine, shortening, mayonnaise) are saturated—generally with hydrogen.

Q. How would it be if I took the cod liver oil after midnight? I always wake up during the night.

A. That's a good plan. Simply make sure that you haven't eaten anything for approximately four hours.

Now you know the type of letters I receive, and the wide range of questions which I answer. Let me hear from you. I'm as close as your nearest mailbox.

CHAPTER XVI

Send Edible Oils To Your Joints
. . . Not Your Liver!

As you struggle to overcome the aching pains of arthritis, there is one organ in your body which will decide your fate.

The potential "villain" is reddish-brown in color, it weighs about 3½ pounds, and it sits astride your small intestine. The liver is sometimes called "the pantry" of the human anatomy . . . because it gobbles up the choicest particles of our food, and stores them for its own use. Your liver can "rob" your system of essential dietary oils—which are so badly needed by your arthritic joints.

The purpose of this chapter is to explain one way you can "by-pass" your liver . . . how you can save the edible oils and utilize them as lubrication.

Cod liver oil, when emulsified and taken on an empty stomach, can be assimilated so that 90% of the oil *shuttles around the liver.* It does not travel *to* the liver via the portal vein.

In contrast, let's compare the effect of edible oils. (I refer to vegetable oils in your salad, or the fats of red meat or fish.) I maintain that with these oils, the most you can deliver to the tissues, eyes, ears and joints is only 65% to 75%. The liver "steals" the rest.

Even worse, if you drink ice-cold beverages or carbonated soda pop with your meals, oil delivery will be reduced to only 5% or 10%.

Perhaps you have read and fully understand the facts about digestion (page 30) and the process of "osmosis" (page 59). Let's assume that you have also selected the right foods, from the list on page 57. All these efforts on your part could be wasted, if you make mistakes in your kitchen. To prevent errors, read and remember the next few paragraphs:

CORRECT COOKING TECHNIQUES ... HOW TO PREPARE FOODS
so you don't destroy the most valuable oils!

The first and foremost suggestion is: "Never use a microwave oven!" The high temperatures are too hot ... the oven incinerates your food, burns away the most important elements. You will destroy the very enzymes, minerals, and vitamins that your body needs most.

Frying is another detrimental method, which I seldom condone. When oil is heated beyond 355 degrees—and a crusty surface forms on fried foods— then your stomach has to use more hydrochloric acid to break down the food. Your body has to supply more lipase from the pancreas to make digestion possible.

Why hasten the wear and tear on your pancreas? Eating too many fried foods makes you more vulnerable to the growth of gallstones.

Now, let's consider the better ways to cook ...

THE WRONG WAY

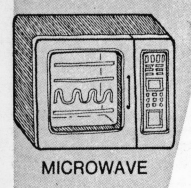

MICROWAVE

THE RIGHT WAY

WATERLESS
COOKING
OR
STEAMING

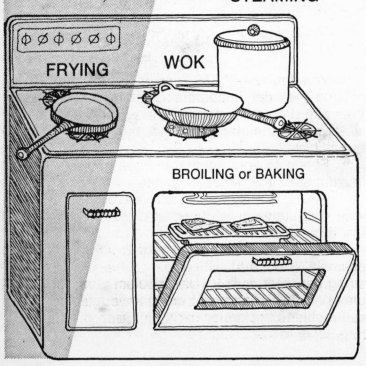

FRYING

WOK

BROILING or BAKING

Broiling is one mode of cooking that I do favor highly. It is more healthful to broil a chicken for 15 to 20 minutes—rather than baking it for an hour.

Always avoid the tendency to "overcook" your foods.

Oven baking should be done at a low temperature . . . just leave the food in the oven for a longer period of time.

Whether broiling or baking, your food should be at room temperature before you start. Defrost, then wait awhile before cooking.

By all means, use a wok whenever you wish. The growing popularity of wok cooking is a trend that I welcome. In this method of preparing foods, you are apt to use more vegetables. That's a dietary plus, any day.

Vegetables—cooked in a wok, for a short length of time—do not become soggy and water-logged. Your aim should be to eat *fresh vegetables* while they are firm and crunchy. One advantage is that you gain more fiber content in your diet.

Steaming your vegetables is a good idea. Very few nutrients will be lost.

Better still, try waterless cooking. This will give your vegetables great flavor at mealtime. Here are a few tips on how it's done:

First, cover the bottom of a pan with diced onions. Next, add some sliced vegetables—like string beans or carrots. Use medium heat, for a minute or so. Then add faster cooking vegetables, which can include zucchini or cabbage. Turn the temperature down to low.

In this example of waterless cooking, the onions should brown lightly, adding delicious flavor to the vegetables. You'll find that the vegetables release enough moisture to steam themselves. Serve this type of food often. It's crispy, better tasting, and best for your health.

MY MENUS, IN CHAPTER XI, CAN BE INTER-CHANGED

You can serve the luncheon foods at dinnertime, or switch any of the dishes within the daily schedule.

The menus are designed for people of all ages. They are beneficial for young and old alike.

Some days you may be in a hurry, and you want to prepare a fast meal. Here are four suggestions, devised with speed in mind:

1. Dip some chicken or fish in egg and bran. Then, bake it.
2. Prepare a quick liquid meal, in a blender.
3. Toast a corn tortilla, topped with Jalapeno cheese.
4. Serve some pita bread, heated and filled with little patties of Falafel mix. (Falafel mix is now available in many grocery stores.)

I have already emphasized the value of having plenty of green vegetables in your daily diet. Let me add that I also favor sprouts. To maintain good health, we all must eat *living plants.* One partial answer is to start your own indoor sprout garden.

It matters not whether you use beans, or alfalfa seeds, or sunflower seeds . . . sprouts are good for you. Check your supermarket, the produce section.

When preparing foods you can often use *your own favorite recipes.* You are not obligated to follow the recipes which I offered on pages 131 through 139. You can *convert* your own recipes, by *substituting more healthful ingredients.* Here is a guide:

YOUR USUAL INGREDIENT	THE RECOMMENDED SUBSTITUTE
1 cup flour............................	Instead, use slightly less than a cup of whole wheat or unbleached pastry flour.
1 cup sugar.........................	¾ cup of honey, plus 4 tablespoons of flour.
1 cup butter........................	¾ cup of unsaturated cold-pressed oil.
1 oz. chocolate...................	3 tablespoons of carob, plus 1 tablespoon of water, plus 1 tablespoon of cold-pressed oil.
3 T. of cocoa......................	4 tablespoons of carob, plus 1 teaspoon of cold-pressed oil, during baking.

SOME FIGHTING WORDS . . . ABOUT ALUMINUM COOKWARE

Throw away those pots and pans! If they are made of aluminum, beware of those cooking utensils. They are a very real threat to your health.

Aluminum poisoning can start in your kitchen . . . it can travel throughout your body, complicate your arthritis, and then damage your brain.

Medical researchers recently performed autopsies on victims of Alzheimer's disease. They found that these patients had about *four times the normal amount of aluminum in their brains.*

This week, I discussed the dangers of aluminum poisoning with an expert, Dr. H. Richard Casdorph.

Dr. Casdorph completed his extensive training in cardiovascular diseases by serving on the staff at the Mayo Clinic. He is the author of more than 50 medical papers, and one of his recent articles is a scientific analysis on the causes of Alzheimer's disease. As a physician, he is currently associated with the Long Beach Community Hospital.

I asked Dr. Casdorph to explain his views on aluminum. He replied, most emphatically:

"I tell people that if they cook with aluminum pots and pans, it may end up in their brain."

Dr. Casdorph offered proof of this frightening fact, by citing research work which is now being done at the University of Toronto. Doctors, in Canada, have discovered alarming amounts of aluminum in the brains of their senile patients.

(I'll quote Dr. Casdorph again, later in this book, in Chapter XVIII. That's where I will devote considerable space to the topic of Alzheimer's.)

Every arthritic should be especially careful to avoid aluminum poisoning. Many related illnesses can be caused, unless your body maintains low levels of aluminum. For example, here is a warning which was published by the Lee Foundation of Nutritional Research in Milwaukee. They stated:

"Such serious disorders as ulcers of the stomach and duodenum, cardiovascular disease, heart failure, obesity and varying degrees of paralysis of the autonomic nervous system appear to be definite consequences of aluminum poisoning."

Take preventive measures, now. I did.

I wondered and worried whether my own body was absorbing too much aluminum. So, I took action . . . to find out!

Did you know that any person can determine the exact level of aluminum in their system, by taking a very simple test? Just send a sample of your hair to a qualified laboratory. Hair analysis has become a recognized science. It is a diagnostic method which I have tried, and I recommend it as being reliable.

In my case, I sent a few strands of my hair to the Analytical Research Labs in Phoenix, Arizona. (There are many such companies, located throughout the United States. By studying the elements in your hair, they can determine the ratios of calcium, zinc, sodium, lead, iron, potassium, etc., which currently exist in your body.)

The first examination of my hair took place (in Phoenix) more than a year ago. Dr. Paul Eck, owner of the laboratory, conducted the research . . . and my particular interest was in the *aluminum* count which would register on his elaborate equipment.

Dr. Eck placed my hair sample in a test tube

filled with perchloride acid. The container was then set on a carousel and spun through an atomic absorbtion spectophotometer. This machine instantly measured, in milligrams per cent, the different elements found in my hair.

My reading—for aluminum—was .90 and was within the "safe" range. Doctors have determined that there is no cause for concern until a person shows a reading of 1.5 or 2.0 in regard to aluminum.

This story—about my personal experience with hair analysis—has an even happier ending. I decided to pay close attention to the way my foods were being cooked. I became "aluminum conscious" for the sake of my health.

Five months later, I sent a second sample of my hair to the same laboratory. The new reading was lower than ever. It's down to .60 and I'll make sure the reduction continues!

THE DEBATE RAGES ON . . . CAN COOKWARE AFFECT YOUR FOOD?

Many voices insist that kitchen utensils *are* a factor. I suggest that everyone should read a classic publication called "The Story of Aluminum Poisoning." (It is a monograph, available through Nutri-Books in Denver, Colorado.) The authors present some excellent arguments, facts you can't ignore. For example:

They cite a test where two quarts of water were boiled in an aluminum pan. An equal amount of water was also boiled in a stainless steel pan. Then, the water was cooled—and some goldfish were placed in each pan.

In six hours the goldfish in the aluminum pan were dead. The other fish were still alive.

You can conduct your own experiments. If you boil cabbage in an aluminum pot, the vessel turns black. There's a chemical reaction.

Boil cherries or grapes in an aluminum pan. If you allow them to stand in the pan for 12 hours, take a good look at what happens. Little pits or holes will be found in the pan!

A HIGHLY-RESPECTED DENTIST JOINS THE FIGHT . . .

His words about aluminum couldn't be stronger. From his office in Maryland, Dr. Arthur F. Furman says this:

"All people must make a concentrated effort to avoid additional contamination of their bodies by this ubiquitous metal."

Dr. Furman's opinion carries real weight. He is a member of the American Dental Association, and is Chief of the Department of Dentistry at Clinton Community Hospital. His reputation is worldwide, and he has served as President of the International Academy of Medical Preventics.

I talked with Dr. Furman, recently, to hear his current position on this matter. He said:

"I urge my patients to throw away their aluminum cookware and never store food overnight in an aluminum container."

So, what shall I tell the readers of this book? What are the best alternatives? Dr. Furman and I both agreed that in your kitchen you should always use the following utensils:

COOK WITH . . .

Stainless steel
Pyrex
Enamelware
Earthenware
Cast iron
Dutch ovens

If you're a mother—teaching your daughter to cook—let her read this book. Then, she can stay healthy. She can *prevent* the illnesses of middle age.

CHAPTER XVII

Health Problems To Watch For At The Age Of 40

Most of my readers are middle-aged. Perhaps you are enjoying those wonderful years . . . the midway mark in your lifetime.

If you feel youthful and healthy, that's all that counts. Forget about birthdays, don't add them up and become depressed.

I often smile when a person tries to hide their age. What's wrong with being 40 . . . if you're hale and hearty? I know vibrant, cheerful people who are twice that age.

Sure, on some days you may feel a bit fatigued. But you can bounce back. Live life to its fullest. You can even become a sexy senior citizen.

Bob Hope, Cary Grant, George Burns . . . they all found the formula for happiness in their later years. So did Lucille Ball, Helen Hayes, and other ladies.

You may be concerned about your future health. Perhaps you are experiencing some early symptoms, a few minor aches and pains which worry you. Let me devote this chapter to some optimistic news. You can prevent many illnesses, if you recognize the first warning signs, and take some simple steps to protect your stamina.

Here's the truth about your life expectancy . . .

Did you know that everyone could live to the age of 120?

The human body is designed to last six times the maturity of your bones. Your bones mature at age 20. (That's when you stop growing in height.) And medical science says that your bodily organs should last 120 years. Anthropologists and gerontologists (doctors who study the aging process) all agree on this fact.

That's an ideal attitude to keep in mind: if you are considered to be "old" at 120, then you are still "middle-aged" on your 60th birthday!

I told this story, half-humorously, during a radio broadcast. A lady listener didn't quite believe it. She was approaching 40, and already her health was deteriorating. I tried to encourage her, lift her spirits.

(Incidentally, the broadcast was originating from WBZ in Boston. This clear channel station, part of the ABC network, is heard throughout New England and all along the Atlantic coast. I had been invited to discuss nutrition. The talk show host was Larry Glick, who has been featured on WBZ for more than 15 years.)

One of the incoming phone calls, during that program, was from this worried lady. Her name was Elizabeth. She reported that she had several symptoms of "middle age"—and I immediately questioned her about her daily diet.

ALEXANDER: Do you wear glasses now?
ELIZBETH: Yes, I do.

ALEXANDER: What beverages have you been drinking?
ELIZABETH: Well, I drink grapefruit juice, all the time.

I explained to Elizabeth that failing eyesight is often caused by consuming acidic fruit juices. Too much carbonic acid travels into the fundus vein of the eye. The costly result is a trip to an optometrist—to be fitted for glasses.

ALEXANDER: Is your hair changing color at all?
ELIZABETH: My hair used to be auburn-colored. Now, it's black.

Perhaps I was able to warn Elizabeth in time. Before her hair turned *grey!* Acid—in fruit juices and soda pop—kills the tyrosinase pigment meant for your hair. (This substance is normally manufactured in the intestinal villi.)

Unless your digestive system is delivering sufficient tyrosinase to the marrow of your hair, color manufacturing stops. Simultaneously, air bubbles will develop in the marrow and *your hair will turn grey or white!*

Signposts of "middle age"—like the weakening of eyesight and the advent of grey hair—are not the end of the world. Most adults can tolerate a few of these minor problems. However, when you reach your middle years, beware of more serious symptoms which could signal your need for real medical care.

If your skin becomes afflicted, in any way, you should take immediate steps and seek prompt advice from a doctor. A complete physical examination, done in time, may save you from dermatitis or psoriasis.

When your skin dries out, you'll know it. First, there's the itching, then the hideous red rash. Worst of all, in psoriasis, you develop patches of scaly skin . . . and it can spread from your hands to your face, chest, and legs.

A typical victim was that lady, in Boston. During the broadcast, she sounded desperate:

ELIZABETH: I heard you say something about cod liver oil helping psoriasis. I have a very serious case . . . and I've tried everything. I've had the ultra-violet treatment, and——

ALEXANDER: Here's what you have to do . . . if you want to have a beautiful skin, without the psoriasis.

It may take three to six months to get well. But you're going to have to mix the cod liver oil with milk, rather than with orange juice. Because you are sensitive to juices.

Cod liver oil will get to the skin and start healing it. It's fantastic for psoriasis, eczema, and will help stop the skin from wrinkling.

ELIZABETH: Great! Okay, thank you. I'm really going to try that . . . and I'll let you know.

For years, I have recommended this same approach. It has a record of proven success against psoriasis.

PUBLISHER'S NOTE: The broadcast on Radio Station WBZ was recorded. Due to limited space, the quotations from that program were edited and condensed.

I shall offer indisputable evidence, throughout this chapter, that people can recover from psoriasis by correcting their eating habits. I'll relate some actual case histories, with facts on how they repaired their damaged skin.

Psoriasis deserves space in this book, because the ailment has become increasingly prevalent among arthritics everywhere. Across America, this disease torments more than 3,000,000 victims!

Unfortunately, 11% of all rheumatoid arthritics also have psoriasis. So, let's discuss the problem in greater detail, and warn you about the consequences.

PSORIASIS . . . THE UGLY PRELUDE TO PSORIATIC ARTHRITIS

By definition, psoriasis is "a chronic, hereditary, recurrent dermatosis—marked by vivid red macules, papules, or plaques covered with silver lamellated scales."

Does that sound frightening? Well, the news gets worse. Very often, victims of psoriasis then develop painfully inflamed terminal interphalangeal joints. Their fingers become swollen and stiff. They have contracted *psoriatic arthritis.*

If you notice pain or swelling in the first joint of your finger (near the fingernail), chances are you have this very common type of arthritis. The saddest part of this story is that *you could have prevented this sickness.* Improper diet caused your psoriatic agony!

I can offer hope. The course of this illness can be reversed. To learn how, let's visit Texas . . .

There's a man you should meet, a real person who now makes his home in the town of Wharton, Texas. He is living proof that psoriasis can be conquered.

His story begins when he was still a teenager. He was attending Abilene Christian College, when his skin suddenly erupted with a severe case of psoriasis.

The year was 1975, and he happened to see me when I appeared on a television talk show at KPRC-TV in Houston. I mentioned how my diet was successful against skin ailments. So, the student contacted me—and we revised his eating habits. (Like many college students, he was consuming too many soft drinks and hamburgers. Junk food caused his system to revolt!) Psoriasis was polluting his face, scalp, chest . . . the rash was covering him, everywhere, except for the palms of his hands and the soles of his feet.

I heard from the young man again, four years later, in 1979. Let me quote, from his letter to me:

"Dale assured me that by following his dietary advice, I could rid myself of this disease. Within six months his predictions had come true.

Today, I still follow Dale's dietary program. I am convinced of its effectiveness. And, although I am not trained in medicine, I can see a direct correlation between what I eat and the condition of my skin.

I am greatly indebted to Dale. His untiring efforts in the field of nutrition, and his deep concern for others, were the cause of my recovery.

I have told others about this diet, with varying results. Those who have tried it have obtained the same favorable results. Others chose not to try the diet, and are in the same condition they were earlier. I urge others suffering from this affliction to try this diet."

Signed: W.W
Wharton, Texas

Letters, like that one, are a joy to receive. Through the years, people from across America have written to me. In some cases, we have become life-long friends.

For example, that young Texan talks with me by telephone—reporting his continued good health. (He is now married, with two children, and he teaches school near Houston.) Most important, his psoriasis has been defeated, permanently. *Ten years have passed,* so nobody can claim that this was temporary remission.

A NATIONAL ORGANIZATION WILL NOW FIGHT PSORIASIS

This illness has become so widespread—with more than 3,000,000 victims in the United States—something had to be done.

I'm glad to report that a special headquarters
has been set up to help expand scientific research on
this one disease. The *National Psoriasis Foundation*
is already in action. You can write to them, for the latest information you need . . . address your letter to
the Foundation, in Portland, Oregon. Zip code
97221.

From them, I asked for a current report on the
types of therapy which are now available to the public. They'll send you a detailed description——citing
the advantages and disadvantages of UVB (ultra-violet light treatments), the validity of PUVA (which utilizes the psoralen drug) and other possible remedies.

I'm now a member of the National Psoriasis
Foundation, and I shall support their goals. They say
that psoriasis may be caused by some type of bio-
chemical stimulus that triggers abnormal cell growth.

I agree with that theory. They state it, quite
clearly: "A normal skin cell matures in 28 to 30 days.
In psoriasis, cells move to the top of the skin in three
days. The excessive skin cells that are produced
"heap up" and form the elevated, red, scaly patches
that characterize psoriasis.

"The white scale that covers the red patch is
composed of dead cells that are continually being
cast off. The redness of the patches is caused by the
increased blood supply necessary to feed this area of
dividing skin cells."

That description fits, very accurately . . . and I
see that skin condition in scores of people who attend
my lectures. My mail constantly includes letters on

the topic of psoriasis. Right now, as I write this chapter, a man in Glendale is recovering from a bad case of psoriasis—thanks to the dietary measures he has taken.

His success story, his victory over this illness, took place very rapidly. (You might be interested to know that, as of today, it has taken me nine months to write this book manuscript. During that same period of time, this gentleman with psoriasis has had some dramatic things happen in his life.)

As an inspiration to others, here's a complete report on his case history . . .

I was contacted by this man, just a few months ago. He is 44 years old and is District Manager of an electronics company, here in California.

Psoriasis had spread across his chest so badly that he was shedding silvery scales of skin.

By analyzing his daily diet, this man quickly realized his errors. He has been drinking a variety of acidic fruit juices—but the real culprit was ice cream. For years, he had consumed copious amounts of ice cream—a habit he now regrets.

He revised his choice of foods, and began to take cod liver oil. Mixing it with milk, as the proper emulsifier.

The result? He tells it best, in his own words:

"After reading your book, I am compelled to write to you.

I have not only suffered from a receding hairline but a psoriasis condition which had been diagnosed as incurable by several doctors over the past 20 years. From a medical standpoint, it was stated that the best I could hope for was to control this condition.

After following the diet outlined in your book for a period of 90 days, I have noticed my skin condition go through a remarkable change. The red sores and bleeding centers have turned to small pink ones with white centers. I know a definite cure is on it's way at last!

To read a book and have these results is close to a divine healing. I trust that others will read your book and follow your diet program and enjoy the new experience that I have with a healthy body.

Sincerely yours,
Mr. J. V.
Glendale, Ca.

When I received that letter, recently, it made my day! Because it proved, once again, that a person can gain better health—without the use of drugs. Why subject yourself to oral psoralen and ultra-violet light? The best road to recovery is via *nutrition*.

ARTHRITIS IS CAUSED BY "WEAR AND TEAR" ON YOUR JOINTS—THAT THEORY IS NOT TRUE! HERE ARE THE REASONS WHY . . .

Too many arthritics have been told that their aches and pains are just part of "growing older"—as though the process of aging is "wearing out" their bodily joints. "Expect some pain, and learn to live with it."

Such a diagnosis is wrong. And don't let anyone blame your arthritis on some "job related" condition. Your occupation, no matter how hard you work, will not "wear out" your joints—if you are eating nutritious foods.

Time and again, whenever I meet with newspaper reporters or magazine writers, they always seem to ask about the same topic. I recall, for example, that the editors of "Healthview Newsletter" pursued this line of questioning. I quoted some of that interview, in Chapter II. On this matter, they minced no words. They demanded the truth:

HEALTHVIEW NEWSLETTER: What about the wear and tear theory?

ALEXANDER: The wear and tear theory states that osteoarthritis can be caused by overactivity in work or exercise. It's said this wears out the cushion of cartilage at the end of the bones.

This theory leaves much to be desired. For instance, for every million persons supposedly suffering from wear and tear arthritis, there are ten million people, of the same age, doing similar work, who do not have it. Why? Because they have the proper lubricating fluid in their joints.

The wear and tear theory was refuted many years ago by Dr. E.F. Rosenberg. (He reported his findings as far back as 1949, in the July issue of the *Journal of the American Medical Association*.) Dr. Rosenberg made the following points:

1. Osteoarthritis of the fingers involves only the end joints. Why isn't the whole finger affected, since all the joints are used equally?
2. Only one hip becomes afflicted. Yet, throughout the years, both hips were used equally.
3. Sedentary workers are often victims of osteoarthritis—without any signs of mechanical or physical wear on their skeletal structures.

In short, the theory just doesn't hold up.

CAN THE CLIMATE AND BAD WEATHER AFFECT YOUR ARTHRITIS?

This notion is false. Weather does not cause arthritis. If geography were really the answer, why are there arthritics in sunny Florida as well as in the snow-covered mountains of Montana?

HEALTHVIEW NEWSLETTER: But don't arthritics feel worse when the weather is damp?

ALEXANDER: That's quite true. However, is the dampness the true cause of the problem? Or is it just irritating poorly lubricated joints already weakened by friction? If weather were really the cause, then everyone would have arthritis during damp weather. But they don't.

Moreover, many arthritics who were sensitive to weather write and tell me that after cod liver oil, it no longer affects them.

For example, I got a letter from a pilot with

Delta Air Lines. He had suffered from inflammation and stiffness in his wrist. Considering his occupation, it was a serious matter. In his letter, he wrote:

"After having been on the cod liver oil program for about three months, I'm hardly aware of any discomfort at all, even on cold, damp days."

When an intelligent reader, like that airlines pilot, reports that my dietary formula has possibly solved a health problem, I feel greatly rewarded. Inspired, I work harder than ever . . . trying to spread the good news, so millions of people can benefit.

I give more lectures, more interviews. To every audience, I keep repeating the same basic message: *Proper foods and eating habits can enhance or increase the quality of synovial fluid in arthritic joints.*

These are the main facts I gave, when I talked with the "Healthview" editors. I also warned them against drinking oil-free liquids with their meals.

(For you, the reader of this book, I'll emphasize this crucial concept by means of a picture. Note, and remember, the Illustration on the next page.)

While those editors were interrogating me, I told them to avoid drinking water, tea or coffee at mealtime. They sounded distressed:

HEALTHVIEW NEWSLETTER: What's so bad about that?
ALEXANDER: When you eat a meal, the food is broken down into minute oily particles and mixed with the stomach juices. The heat in the stomach changes any fats in the food into tiny oily globules.

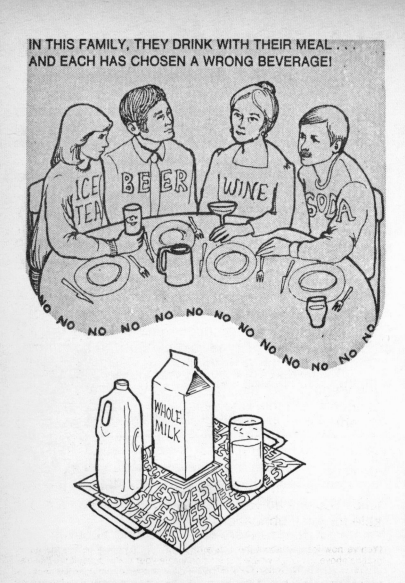

**THEY WOULD BE MUCH WISER TO ENJOY
WHOLE MILK AT MEALTIME!**

If you don't drink liquids, here's what happens . . .

The tiny oily globules (about half of them) are collected by something called the cisterna chyli. This is a passageway leading out of the stomach and emptying eventually into the bloodstream.

The oily globules travel along this passageway, get to the bloodstream and are transported to the joints. The remaining oils will travel on and eventually enter the portal vein and go to the liver.

However, if you drink an oil-free beverage with your meal, the picture changes. The beverage causes the oil globules to rupture into one large pool. Now, only about 20% of them can enter the cisterna chyli, bypass the liver, and go directly to the joints. The other 80% go on to the portal vein. They end up in the liver, which uses them for energy and other metabolic purposes——not as lubricants.

If you want your dietary oils to act as lubricants, you've got to get them to bypass your liver. The way to accomplish this is to avoid all mealtime beverages, except milk or soups. These two beverages cause no problems because they already contain tiny particles of oil. Hence they don't disturb the globules in the stomach.

So, to sum up, avoid oil-free beverages at mealtime. You will actually triple the amount of oils available for joint lubrication.

(You've now learned about the "cisterna chyli" . . . as described in the paragraphs above. To know where it is located inside your body, consult the Illustration on page 245. Find the thoracic duct. Follow it down, from near the neck, to where it disappears behind the stomach. Right there——in the lumbar region behind the stomach——is your *cisterna chyli*. Actually, it is a dilated part of the thoracic duct.)

"TELEVISION" REMEDIES . . . PILLS BEING PUSHED ON TV

There are so many products being advertised, we are totally confused and annoyed. Arthritics are now being bombarded by TV commercials. The announcers all make the same claim: "Relief from pain! Just try our new capsule . . . our medicine is *best!*"

When I lecture to an audience these days, I can count on hearing questions about Ecotrin, Ascriptin, Advil, etc.

I never discuss the merits of these products, nor compare one against the other. Swallowing pills—even old-time favorites like Bufferin, Excedrin and Aspirin—is not the way to defeat arthritis. In my opinion, they are just stop-gap measures. Temporary solutions to a chronic illness.

Through the years, I have warned my readers that any drug can become addictive or dangerous. Take too many aspirin, too often, and before long you might become a victim of peptic ulcers.

It is quite obvious that I am "anti-drugs" . . . and there are many good reasons for my negative vote. I summarized my attitude, in Chapter V of this book.

I must remind you that certain drugs may bring temporary relief for rheumatoid arthritis—yet they have no effect at all on osteoarthritic symptoms. Synthetic cortisone is one example . . . it is useless against knobby fingers or frozen shoulders.

May I also emphasize that I am not a solo voice when I find fault with prescription drugs. Among the leading physicians who are opposed to drug therapy is Doctor Robert Mendelsohn of Chicago.

At the University of Illinois, Dr. Mendelsohn served on the faculty. He has been National Medical Director for "Project Head Start"—and Chairman of the Medical Licensing Committee for the State of Illinois. Therefore, I value his opinions when he speaks out *against* drug therapy for arthritics.

I have discussed the drug problem with him, and we are in complete agreement. Dr. Mendelsohn and I have known each other for years. You might recognize him, from his frequent appearances on network television. He has twice been a guest on "The Phil Donahue Show" . . . and his views have sparked lively debate.

Warner Books, a division of the giant Warner Communications Company, believes in Dr. Mendelsohn. They published the soft-cover version of his famous book. It is entitled: "Confessions of a Medical Heretic."

Let me quote just a few sentences from that book. Dr. Mendelsohn is reporting how the drug companies have spared neither time nor money in rushing their arthritis "cures" to the marketplace. He then says . . .

"Just reading the information supplied *by the manufacturer* of Butazolidin alka, and thinking that your doctor actually is prescribing the stuff to you is enough to make you ill: 'This is a potent drug; its misuse can lead to serious results. Cases of leukemia have been reported in patients with a history of short and long term therapy. The majority of the patients were over forty.' If you read further you find that your doctor is setting you up for a possible 92 adverse reactions, including headaches, vertigo, coma, hypertension, retinal hemorrhage, and hepatitis.''

Bravo! I applaud Dr. Mendelsohn. He certainly has intestinal fortitude. He tells it like it is!

LECITHIN. SHOULD ARTHRITICS "BUY" THIS PRODUCT?

Should you purchase extracted lecithin and use it to supplement your daily diet? That's a question asked by many arthritics—because lecithin is being heavily advertised as an effective weapon to relieve rheumatic pains.

Don't buy this idea—about the healing qualities of lecithin—until you read the next few paragraphs.

I have certain reservations about lecithin, and I shall state them honestly. Research efforts are now underway, and some companies are already manufacturing "lecithin" tablets or pills. I have my doubts whether such capsules, taken orally, can accomplish results for arthritics.

On the other hand, I do favor the daily use

of "powdered" lecithin—which is already available in health food stores.

What *is* lecithin? Your own body produces this substance, naturally. It is a protein . . . some types of lecithin are found in various tissues of your body and in your blood.

Lecithin is a raw material which helps your liver to synthesize the foods you eat. In fact, some foods actually contain lecithin. Soy beans and egg yolk, for example, are sources of this protein.

For years, I have augmented my diet with small quantities of lecithin. By the teaspoonful.

For arthritics, I have already recommended that lecithin should be included in your dietary program. For instance, on page 126 of this book, you will note that lecithin is one of the crucial ingredients in my Special Health Drink.

My confidence in the value of lecithin dates back many years. I learned that lecithin contains a helpful supply of B-complex vitamins, like choline.

Scientists have proved that *choline* can help reduce lesions. (In arthritis—when cartilages or the linings of the joints start to degenerate—lesions begin to appear.)

I studied medical papers which were published by Dr. Charles H. Best. He was the co-discoverer of insulin, in the battle against diabetes.

Dr. Best conducted many experiments, trying new diets on groups of rats. In one series of tests, he fed 20 rats a choline-deficient diet. Soon, 15 of the rats developed hemorrhagic kidney lesions and cardiac problems. He concluded that any diet for humans must contain adequate amounts of choline.

The importance of choline—and the true value of lecithin—are now being emphasized as the medical world seeks a cure for Alzheimer's disease. (I give my findings about Alzheimer's later in this book. See Chapter XVIII).

Lecithin is acquiring a worldwide reputation as a key factor in restoring health. For example, let me tell you about a recent conference which was held in Vienna, Austria. Doctors, biochemists, and nutrition researchers from 15 different countries were present.

The seminar continued for three days. It was the Third International Symposium on Alzheimer's disease.

I was invited to participate. I booked a flight from Los Angeles and flew to Austria . . . because this conference would consolidate the latest progress being made in medical research.

Arriving in Vienna, I met colleagues from Japan, Italy, the Scandinavian countries—all of us with the same goal. Defeat the curse of Alzheimer's disease!

There was much discussion about dietary methods, about lecithin, and about the importance of choline. Some pharmacologists who were present now want to synthesize choline in test tubes. I hope they will decide to extract *natural choline* from soy beans.

Meanwhile, I shall continue to recommend that all arthritics should consider lecithin, carefully. It has beneficial qualities . . . but use it sparingly, with common sense.

WILL YOUR SEX LIFE IMPROVE . . . AFTER AGE 40?

Your sexual activity can increase—and be far more enjoyable in the years ahead—if you just read these next few paragraphs.

I am not going to write "advice for the lovelorn" . . . and this book will not describe any new positions for more erotic sex. However, I do intend to reveal some facts that can increase your sexual pleasure, no matter what your age.

A healthy sex life can be yours, if you will take better care of certain glands in your body.

I'll hazard a guess that 9 out of 10 women have never even heard of their Bartholin glands.

Most men, by the same token, know nothing about their Tyson gland—couldn't find it if they tried.

Yet, all those glands play very essential roles during sexual intercourse.

A key element, for performing the sex act, is lubrication. The Bartholin and Tyson glands provide lubrication—not semen—to make insertion far more pleasant. Natural lubrication is best. You won't need gel-like products purchased in stores.

I often wondered why gynecologists do not give their patients enough information about these vital glands. Medical textbooks report that the discovery of the glands was made centuries ago.

Women can be grateful to Dr. Casper Bartholin. He did so much research, back in the year 1655, that the glands were named after him. While he was at work, in his native Denmark, another physician (across the channel, in England) was conducting tests among men. Dr. Edward Tyson was studying a particular gland that could secrete special lubrication during the sex act.

Let's bring this story forward——to the present day. In recent decades, millions of people did read a certain book about sex and marriage. Random House published it. The title was: "Ideal Marriage——Its Physiology and Technique."

In that volume, if you look very closely, there is brief mention of a woman's Bartholin glands. An illustration shows that the two glands are located at the entrance to the vagina.

The Bartholin glands lie, one on each side, on the lateral walls of the vaginal introitus. Their function is described as follows:

"They manufacture a perfectly transparent, thin and very slippery mucus secretion, which, as a rule is only exuded under the influence of sexual stimuli, particularly as a result of *initial psychic excitement*.

"In normal cases, the amount of mucus is just sufficient *for purposes of lubrication of the introitus* vaginae, and, together with similar urethral secretions of the man, enables coitus to be carried out."

(Remarkably, the same function is performed by the Tyson gland in a man. His gland is located in the corona of his penis. A healthy male will secrete the same type of lubrication as his mate.)

HOW TO "AWAKEN" YOUR GLANDS . . . FOR SEXUAL DELIGHT

If you and your partner want better performance, sexually, that's a happy goal. And, by now, you can probably predict the advice I shall offer.

Yes, I'm going to recommend *proper diet* . . . as your best guarantee to stimulate both Bartholin and Tyson glands. After all, we are still talking about the same subject: *lubrication.* The amount of natural lubrication which your body can create depends on what you eat!

'C'mon, Alexander? Next you're going to tell us that cod liver oil is good for our sex life!"

That's right! My research indicates that the Bartholin and Tyson glands require certain nutrients. They need *the same fatty acids* found in cod liver oil!

Every day, these particular glands must receive an adequate supply of essential fatty acids. Feed them——by eating healthful foods, as described in this book. And augment your diet with cod liver oil. Only then will you provide your body with enough linoleic, linolenic and arachidonic acid.

Don't let these glands "dry out"——because that could lead to hospitalization and worse. There's more at stake than just sexual fun and games. If just one Bartholin gland dries up, near your vagina, it could result in cancer.

I hope that the new information, in these few

pages will help lubricate your sex organs. There are better things to do in bed than read a book.

FOR MIDDLE-AGED READERS ... SOME FINAL ADVICE
Facts You Need To Know About LUPUS

There is one insidious ailment—with the short name of "lupus"—which is now sneaking up on thousands of new victims every year.

At all my lectures, someone in the audience is bound to ask questions about this rheumatic illness. They want to learn more about the symptoms—and how they can cope with *systemic lupus erythematosus.*

Women, especially, fear this disease—because it often leaves permanent marks on their faces. Most females feel threatened ... they know that lupus strikes women about 8 to 10 times as often as men.

The facial damage caused by lupus is a red rash, followed by marks which resemble the bite of a wolf.

Lupus means *wolf* ... it's a word taken from the Latin language, which aptly describes the most common symptom of this affliction. After "wolf marks" develop on a victim's face, the rash often progresses down across the nose and into the cheek areas. By then, the markings often appear to be butterfly-shaped.

Don't get the idea that lupus merely affects a

lady's vanity. This is far more than just a cosmetic problem. Lupus can be dangerous and disabling. The symptoms you may experience include muscle aches, swollen glands, nausea and vomiting.

Inflammation often occurs, which can result in kidney problems and pleurisy (an inflammation of the outer coverings of the lungs).

I maintain that lupus is a disorder of the connective tissues. It resembles rheumatoid activity of the same type that occurs in rheumatoid arthritis.

Early signs of lupus can be recognized. You may notice joint pain in your hands, wrists, elbows, knees, or ankles.

Medical science now believes that your body's immune system may hold the key as to what causes lupus. There are three main types of immune cells— all are circulating in your blood and body fluids. Their job is to attack harmful bacteria and viruses.

The subject of autoimmune disease is so vitally important, I shall discuss it in detail later on. (See Chapter XIX)

In the opinion of some, lupus may be related to a lack of protein or factors being present in your thymus gland. Let me report on one series of tests . . .

Dr. Jerry Daniels, at the University of Texas Medical Branch in Galveston, has given thymus hormone to patients with systemic lupus. He and his colleagues believe that it will correct certain immune imbalances.

(Your thymus gland, incidentally, is located in your neck close to the thyroid. Starting in childhood, this gland needs vitamins, minerals, and essential fatty acids in order to develop properly.)

Women, in their child-bearing years, are most susceptible to lupus. It has also been proven that, for some reason, lupus occurs more frequently in blacks and in certain Indian tribes than among whites.

Actually, lupus is now attacking thousands of people, worldwide. I saw the "wolf marks" on great numbers of victims throughout Great Britain.

A special Rheumatology Unit has been established at the Royal Postgraduate Medical School at Hammersmith Hospital in London. More than 72 specialists——doctors from Australia, America, New Zealand, Hong Kong, etc.——have traveled to this hospital to receive advance training for the war against lupus.

Not long ago, to honor these doctors, a noted guest visited the Hammersmith Lupus Unit. Princess Diana toured the wards, personally talking with the bedridden lupus patients.

If a final answer is discovered——a permanent cure for lupus——it may very well come from London, from this outstanding group of dedicated scientists.

I hope this Chapter, which was written for all middle-aged readers, has proved helpful. Next, let's turn to health problems affecting the more elderly . . .

CHAPTER XVIII

Helpful Facts For Senior Citizens with special reports on Alzheimer's Disease and Parkinson's Disease

When you become a bit timeworn and aged, what will be the state of your health? Most people who have arthritis also worry about other afflictions which may disable them during their senior years.

By taking a few precautions, now, you can avoid many ailments as you grow older.

In this chapter, my purpose is to alert you, in advance, about certain symptoms—so you can avert a health catastrophe in the future.

It is quite possible for you to approach old age with a strong body and an alert mind. The decision is yours. When you reach the age of 65, would you rather be agile or fragile?

If you watch your diet—and eat wisely—you can prevent the onslaught of most diseases.

Even the pains of arthritis can be borne more easily than a mental illness like Alzheimer's disease. Complete loss of memory—total senility—is a tragedy we all fear.

I shall discuss Alzheimer's at some length, and

warn you about the dietary mistakes which might cause your brain to degenerate. I believe that arthritics, in particular, need to know these facts . . .

ALZEHIMER'S DISEASE . . . BRAIN DAMAGE, TOTAL SENILITY

The term "Alzheimer's disease" was seldom used, until 10 years ago. People suffered from the illness, but it was not discussed openly.

There seemed to be a certain stigma attached to this affliction. An aged person was displaying feeble-mindedness, loss of memory, embarrassing signs of total senility.

Now, however, the public is more sympathetic—because they understand the symptoms of the Alzheimer syndrome . . . and they realize this disease can strike anyone in their later years.

Currently, this tragic form of intellectual impairment has claimed 1,500,000 victims in the United States. Alzheimer's disease is 14 times more common than multiple sclerosis.

Everyone wonders what causes Alzheimer's. In my opinion, *dryness* is to blame. The same lack of oils that occurs in arthritic joints is also injurious to patients with Alzheimer's. In this case, the dryness is in the sheath or coverings of the nerve tissues in the brain cortex.

The outer layer of the brain, because of dryness, develops an accumulation of abnormal fibers. Under a microscope, these changes appear as a tangle of filaments. These neurofibrillary tangles were first discovered by a German neurologist named Alois Alzheimer.

With these basic facts as background, let us now take a close look at Alzheimer's disease. A large percentage of arthritics eventually succumb to Alzheimers, so let's talk *prevention.*

I believe that the dietary recommendations made in this book will also provide helpful nutrients to forestall Alzheimer's disease.

Nourish the nerve tissues in the brain cortex, with oil-bearing foods . . . that's one way to prevent degenerative brain damage.

Another important step you can take is to seek help from your local chapter of ADRDA. Yes, there is a national organization which you can turn to for advice. It's called the *Alzheimer's Disease and Related Disorders Association.*

You may suspect that some member of your family is slowly developing Alzheimer's. Their memory is failing . . . they show signs of confusion, irritability, restlessness, and agitation.

If you recognize these symptoms, have the person examined by a doctor. Unless you act, now, the victim of Alzheimer's may be headed for serious trouble.

As the illness worsens, the patient will lose judgement, concentration, orientation . . . even their speech may be affected.

A physician can take an electroencephalogram. This may show a general slowing of the brain waves—and could confirm the presence of Alzheimer's.

IS ALUMINUM POISONING A FACTOR IN ALZHEIMER'S?

Yes. There is medical proof to confirm this danger. For example, Dr. David Shore tells of tests, including autopsies: *"The brain aluminum level of Alzheimer's patients is four to six times the levels found in normal brain cells."*

Dr. Shore is a prominent researcher at Saint Elizabeth's Hospital in Washington, D.C. On the West Coast some additional warnings have been issued by Dr. Richard Casdorph. (See page 186.) In an interview—for *Health Freedom News*—he said:

"We are literally swimming in an environment of aluminum. As you may know, aluminum ore comprises 15% of the earth's crust.

"Because of industrial pollution, so-called acid rain is increasing the amount of aluminum that dissolves in rain water, which becomes our drinking water.

"We are being infused with aluminum. It is used commercially in baking powders, underarm deodorants and antacids."

According to Trace Minerals Systems of Alexandria, Virginia—which is a leading laboratory in the field of hair analysis—more and more people are becoming afflicted with toxic levels of aluminum. The problem is almost endemic across America.

We are discussing an illness which is also known as "senile dementia" . . . and senior adults have good reason to fear this affliction. Alzheimer's disease causes 60,000 to 90,000 deaths annually!

Two doctors, at the Massachusetts Institute of Technology, are doing some of the best research on the problem of Alzheimer's. They are a married couple—Dr. Richard Wurtman and Dr. Judith Wurtman. Quite recently, they edited a five-book publication. It is entitled "Nutrition and the Brain"—and I consider it a classic work.

Next, a news item from *The Washington Post* . . .

When it comes to investigative reporting, the foremost newspaper in our nation is *The Washington Post*. Read their comment, published recently:

"Aluminum, one of the most common elements on earth and long thought to be harmless, also may be implicated in several forms of human brain degeneration, particularly Alzheimer's disease."

They based this statement on recent findings made by scientists at Cornell University, Dartmouth College, and the University of Vermont. Researchers at these institutions found aluminum in high-altitude streams—in sufficient concentrations to be toxic to fish and aquatic life, and apparently damaging to trees and plants.

"The Post" went on to say that there is *"a gath-*

ering consensus that acid rain's apparent tendency to mobilize aluminum poses a potential public health problem.''

Doctors already know that the human body stores its highest concentrations of aluminum in the lungs, liver, thyroid and brain. Antacid tablets, which we Americans consume by the millions, contain aluminum hydroxide gel. This habit could reduce your blood phosphate level.

In a person with low blood phosphate, their bones begin to dissolve, their muscles ache and are extremely weak.

Perhaps these facts have given you some helpful knowledge about Alzheimer's disease. For more information, contact the National Institute on Aging, or the National Institute of Health, in Bethesda, Md.

PARKINSON'S DISEASE . . . TREMBLING LIMBS, AND DEMENTIA

There once was a friendly old man, an actor and comedian named Ed Wynn. (Remember? He was ''The Texaco Fire Chief'' in the early days of television.)

In his later years, whenever Ed Wynn appeared on TV, we watched with compassion. Because his hands were trembling, he walked hesitantly, and he spoke with great difficulty. Ed Wynn was a victim of Parkinson's disease.

The staggering truth is that 1,000,000 people,

throughout the United States, now have this vicious affliction. Every year, more than 50,000 Americans learn they have Parkinson's!

This disease affects both men and women, mostly those who are 40 years of age or older.

Dr. James Parkinson, a London physician, first described this illness. His research was done in the year 1817—and the problem has been growing ever since. Now, in the next few pages, I'll try to give you a current picture on where we stand.

First, you will need to know something about your basal ganglion. In anatomy, the ganglion is a group of nerve cell bodies . . . and we are interested in those which are located next to your brain stem.

Basically, Parkinson's is a brain disease. Some doctors compare it to "hardening of the brain arteries" . . . and a concentrated effort is now underway to find a cure. The National Parkinson Foundation has been established, based in Miami, Florida.

To protect yourself, and your loved ones, you should learn the early symptoms of Parkinson's. There is more involved than just noticing tremors and slowness of movement.

Other manifestations of Parkinson's are easy to identify. Researchers, at the Foundation, have published this list:

1. Victims of Parkinson's have episodes of "freezing"—where they have sudden difficulty in walking. They freeze, particularly in moving through a doorway or in turning.

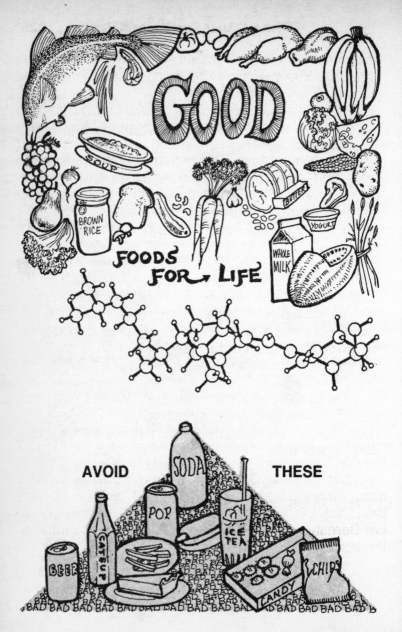

GOOD

FOODS FOR LIFE

SOUP
BROWN RICE
BUTTER
YOGURT
WHOLE MILK

AVOID   THESE

SODA
POP
ICE TEA
KETSUP
BEER
CANDY
CHIPS

BAD BAD BAD BAD BAD BAD BAD BAD BAD BAD BAD BAD B

224

2. They experience dementia, and show a decreased memory for recent events.
3. They exhibit periods of depression.
4. Some patients sweat excessively, and have oily skin. May have visual problems simultaneously.
5. Cramps may occur. Plus a burning sensation in the thighs or legs.
6. Another indication is when the person has low backache, accompanied by poor posture.

If you encounter any of the six symptoms listed above, you should seek a doctor's advice immediately.

The final problem we ought to discuss is speech impairment caused by Parkinson's. This illness often affects the muscles necessary for speech production.

Muscles in the mouth, cheeks, jaw and lips fail to function properly. Rigidity of the facial muscles makes even smiling difficult. The patient may have reduced breath support. This is caused by rigidity of the chest muscles—therefore, the person will have low volume and a weak sounding voice.

As I have indicated, there is now a splendid organization which is actively seeking a cure for Parkinson's. The Foundation, in Miami, will send you detailed booklets if you need more facts.

Bob Hope is Chairman of their Board of Governors. Other members of the Board include Lucille Ball, Dick Clark, Pearl Bailey, Steve Allen and Leonard Bernstein. Quite a group! All dedicated to ending the scourge of Parkinson's.

PROPER DIET CAN HELP . . . DEFEAT DRYNESS AS FIRST STEP

I believe that the same dryness experienced by arthritics is also dangerous to anyone with Parkinson's.

Dryness—in the basal ganglion, next to the brain stem—should be avoided at all costs. Food nutrients are needed to help your brain make acetylcholine. Your diet should supply choline. As one rich source, you should eat more fish.

Lecithin also contains choline (as phosphatidylcholine) . . . so, act accordingly.

Some doctors report that Parkinson's is caused by an oxidative process. To gain a degree of protection, you could try antioxidants . . . such as Vitamins C, E, B-1, B-5, and B-6.

If you can detect this disease early—and seek medical help—the patient can survive for many years.

In addition to trembling fingers and tremors, watch for these signs: the victim develops a stooped position and a slow, shuffling gait. He or she may acquire a diminished facial expression, and may hold arms fixed at the side when walking.

To conclude our discussion about Parkinson's disease, let me simplify the main facts . . .

1. Your brain works because your nerves talk to each other—with chemicals called neuro-transmitters.

2. Neuro-transmitters are manufactured in your body from nutrients in the food you eat.

As scientific research continues, it may well develop that good nutrition is the ultimate answer to Parkinson's.

Why have I devoted so much space in this book to the subject of Parkinson's? Because nearly 5% of all arthritics eventually develop this illness. Let's start working, now, to reduce that figure!

At almost all my lectures, several people in the audience asked questions about Parkinson's disease.

"Is it inherited?" No. There is no medical evidence to indicate that this illness can be passed from generation to generation. Also, the ailment is not considered to be contagious.

"Is exercise advised?" Yes, some doctors do recommend a program of special exercises. To reduce rigidity of muscles, and to prevent atrophy.

"Is any medication available?" That question opens a whole controversy. As you know, I am quite adamant—against the use of drugs. However, some physicians believe that patients with Parkinson's are suffering from a lack of dopamine. To replace this chemical—to stimulate the nerve cells in the brain— the current prescription is usually for L-DOPA.

I'll leave the choice up to you. Improve your diet for permanent relief. Or, it's L-DOPA.

CANCER ARTHRITIS . . . INFLAMMATION, FOLLOWED BY TUMORS

Anyone, after taking a physical examination, is nervous. If the doctor even mentions the word *cancer,* the patient becomes terrified.

So, very few people have been told that they have "cancer arthritis"—the term is seldom used. But the disease exists.

I intend to describe the symptoms, and reveal the history of this illness. Knowledge can keep you forewarned.

Cancer arthritis was really discovered—and was clinically studied—more than 25 years ago. The two doctors, who deserve credit for their research, were associated with a hospital in Copenhagen, Denmark. Dr. Brynjolf Strandberg and Dr. Neils Jarlov reported their findings at the Third International Congress of Physical Medicine, held in Washington, D.C., in 1960.

They conducted their tests, among 53 patients, all of whom were hospitalized. The patients had been diagnosed, previously, as suffering from rheumatoid arthritis.

Dr. Strandberg determined that rheumatoid arthritics often have inflamed joints—and lesions which later developed into tumors.

In these patients, the protein levels of their blood was in disarray. Their alkaline phosphatase level was elevated. Their albumin-globulin ratio was reversed. Normally, they should have had two parts of albumin to one part of globulin. Instead, these "cancer arthritis" patients had the opposite reading.

Stated in more simple language, the early signs of this illness manifest themselves as follows: you might notice swelling, stiffness and restricted movement—first in the small joints of the fingers, then in the toes, foot, elbow, knee, shoulder and hip.

Other symptoms include inflammation and fatigue. As lesions grow worse, they progress toward becoming tumors. Dr. Strandberg concluded: "Rheumatoid arthritis may be the first clinical sign of cancer."

When I learned that cancer and arthritis might be closely related, I began attending conferences to study this combined threat to everyone's health. A dozen years ago, I joined the I.A.C.V.F.—the International Association of Cancer Victims and Friends.

(Later, I was elected Vice President of that organization, and served for three years. I am also a member of the Cancer Control Society. They have 30 chapters, nationwide. This year, I lectured at their 12th annual conference.)

A BELOVED MOVIE STAR DIES . . . FROM CANCER ARTHRITIS

This illness is not something new. For example, several years ago it claimed the life of a famous personality. Rosalind Russell died, in 1976. If you remember some of the newspaper articles, they reported that her death was due to *cancer rheumatoid arthritis.*

While I was writing this book, I contacted the National Cancer Institute. I was seeking their latest recommendations on how to *prevent* cancer. And here's a very interesting development. *They* are suggesting that *proper foods* can protect your health!

"Current evidence suggests that by choosing carefully and eating a well-balanced diet, you may reduce your cancer risk."

They said it, not I. But, naturally, I am in total agreement with their nutritional approach.

Let me quote exactly what they recommend:

"Eat a variety of foods every day. Include fresh fruits and vegetables, especially those high in vitamin A and C . . . such as oranges, grapefruit, nectarines, cantaloupe, and honeydew melons."

(I can only add that you should *eat* these foods, and *chew* them well.)

They go on to say . . . "Choose leafy green and yellow-orange vegetables. Like spinach, kale, sweet potatoes, and carrots, as well as cabbage, cauliflower, broccoli and brussels sprouts.

"Eat foods with fiber, such as whole grain breads and cereals; a variety of raw fruits and vegetables, especially if eaten with the skin; beans, peas, and seeds."

Does all this sound vaguely familiar? Of course it does. You've been reading the same advice, since page one of this book.

To prevent cancer—and cancer arthritis—you can also rely on certain vitamins. The United States Department of Health and Human Services has voiced their favorable opinion about essential vitamins.

In a booklet, prepared in cooperation with the National Institute of Health, they emphasize the role that vitamins should play in your daily diet.

Quoting them, I also agree with these facts . . .

"Scientists have found some relationship between a lack of certain vitamins—A and C—and cancer. For example, diets low in Vitamin A have been linked to cancers of the prostate gland, cervix, skin, bladder, and colon.

"You can get all the vitamins A and C your body can use if you choose two helpings daily from the same fruits and vegetables that are in a balanced diet—dark green vegetables, yellow-orange vegetables, and yellow-orange fruits.

If you are worried about contracting cancer, these past few pages have given you a clear guide on how to minimize your odds. Now, let's turn to another health problem, one which haunts millions of people during their senior years.

HIGH BLOOD PRESSURE . . . THE INVISIBLE DISEASE

You don't even know you have it. This illness gives you no outward signs—no swollen fingers, no painful symptoms to warn you of trouble. High blood pressure can creep up on a person, unnoticed.

Only one third of the people who have this ailment are being treated. And half of those patients don't follow their physician's advice rigorously enough to bring their blood pressure under control.

Because it is essentially painless—until you are felled by a stroke or a heart attack—you tend to ignore your blood pressure. That's a bad gamble!

Sixty million Americans are seven times more likely to have a stroke than their fellow citizens, just because their blood pressure is higher.

Most doctors agree that high blood pressure is usually caused by one of the three s's. *Salt, Stress,* or *Smoking.*

One out of four Americans could really benefit from therapy—their blood pressure has elevated to an unacceptable level.

I shall have much to say, shortly, about sodium in your diet. Basically, the key rule is: "Don't use that salt shaker!"

Most adults, especially elders, now eat about 10 to 12 grams of sodium chloride each day. The sad fact is, your kidneys were created to deal with only *one tenth* of that amount.

In order for your body to excrete the "salt" you will need more water in your system. The salt must be diluted. By the time you become a senior citizen, your body is automatically retaining five or ten pounds of extra water—to aid in the dilution of salt.

Pressure must be exerted, by your own vascular system, to force out the sodium excretion. This may place a burden on your kidneys. The added work causes your blood pressure to soar.

STRESS. DOCTORS NOW CALL IT "HYPERTENSION" . . .

If the patient seems nervous and distraught—causing a rise in blood pressure—it is now popular to blame it all on hypertension.

"Here's a pill, to calm you down." The most common prescriptions, to fight high blood pressure, include Rauwolfia tablets, Reserpine, Aldomet, Adoril, etc. Why? Why do we always turn to *drugs?*

My objection to oral medication is not just a solo crusade. On this matter, my views run parallel with those of Dr. Cleaves Bennett. He is one of the nation's foremost experts on hypertension.

Dr. Bennett began his career in New York State, by graduating from the University of Rochester School of Medicine and Dentistry. After earning his M.D., he became a nephrologist—a physician specializing in kidney diseases.

Most recently, Dr. Bennett wrote an important book. It was published by Doubleday and Company (New York). Speaking forcefully, the title is: *Control Your High Blood Pressure Without Drugs!*

This learned doctor says it quite plainly, in one sentence: *"High blood pressure can and should be controlled by good nutrition, exercise, and stress reduction."*

Dr. Bennett describes high blood pressure as "the silent killer" . . . so heed that warning, now. Damage can be going on inside you, where you can't feel it. Inside your arteries, inside your kidneys, even inside your eyes.

He concludes: "That shortness of breath that stops you when you walk, or wakes you at night, is another sign of blood pressure out of control."

I recommend that you read Dr. Bennett's book. He outlines a 12-week program that attacks the causes of hypertension on three major fronts. The three key answers are: diet modification, stress reduction, and simple but regular exercise.

For added evidence, let's meet another doctor . . .

Dr. Robert Downs practices in Albuquerque, New Mexico. He, too, has done extensive research on many circulatory diseases, including high blood pressure. I have known Dr. Downs for nearly 10 years, and have met with him for conferences about nutrition. As an author, he writes a popular column on health topics.

Dr. Downs received nationwide attention, not long ago, when he discussed garlic as having possible therapeutic value. He was interviewed by a writer from *Bestways* Magazine, which published these facts:

BESTWAYS: What do you use in treating high blood pressure patients?

DR. DOWNS: Garlic works to reduce hypertension. Because of the oil components and chemicals which stimulate a certain prostaglandin in the body to shift the sodium balance out of the cells.

It (garlic) acts as a cellular diuretic and reduces high blood pressure in a mild way. Because of the oil components in the garlic, it inhibits the platelets from aggregating, thins the blood, provides less risk of blood clots and a better blood flow.

I respect Dr. Downs, and I concur with his findings which favor garlic.

Notice that he mentions a *prostaglandin.* That may be a new word for most of my readers. It is a term which is of fundamental importance to all victims of arthritis. You will learn more about prostaglandins in the next chapter—how they may control inflammation and reduce arthritic pain.

Prostaglandins are of such significance to you, let's take a moment to explain what they are. This is the definition, from Dorland's Medical Dictionary:

PROSTAGLANDIN—Any of a group of naturally occurring, chemically related hydroxy fatty acids that stimulate contractility of the uterine and other smooth muscle and *have the ability to lower blood pressure,* regulate acid secretion of the stomach, regulate body temperature and platelet aggregation, *and to control inflammation* and vascular permeability; they also affect the action of certain hormones.

Medical research on prostaglandins is now a major activity in laboratories throughout the world. (See Chapter XX.)

But, right now, let's return to the subject of

plain, ordinary garlic. Is it conceivable that the tiny buds from this strong-smelling plant can actually reduce high blood pressure?

Yes, I agree with Dr. Downs. Garlic can help. Extractions (taken from raw garlic) are available in three forms: capsules, tablets, and liquid garlic.

I believe that the capsules are best. Take them with your food . . . but, remember, don't wash them down with water.

You may find, however, that you need as many as six capsules per day—in order to make some headway in reducing your high blood pressure.

Perhaps a better idea is to eat more raw garlic. Grind it up, into your salads. Just one or two buds of garlic a day. Rub your salad bowl with them. Add garlic, to spice up some of your recipes.

ARTHRITICS HAVE BLOOD SLUDGING . . . POOR CIRCULATION

Most patients with arthritis also find that their circulatory system is not functioning properly. Blood sludge is evident—and that can cause your blood pressure to rise.

To prevent blood sludging, I recommend a diet which is high in magnesium content. This will help to dilate your blood vessels.

Among the best foods—containing magnesium—are legumes, nuts, and whole grains. You can also gain magnesium by eating fish and lean meat.

In these last few pages, I have given you the current thinking about high blood pressure and related ailments. To summarize: SALT is your worst enemy.

To avoid salt, don't eat cold cuts, and don't use salty condiments, like catsup. If you are fighting high blood pressure, *do* drink more water. Have a glass of water ten minutes *before* a meal—or drink it at least three to four hours *after* a meal.

Water will hydrate your system. It will help your body eliminate excess salt, via your kidneys.

This entire chapter has been directed toward senior citizens, older people who are ailing. I could cover many topics. When you age, you become prone to a wide variety of health problems . . . failing eyesight, loss of hearing, insomnia, constipation, etc.

But there is one serious illness which I feel compelled to discuss. Many arthritics simultaneously suffer from diabetes. For several pages, the villain has been salt. Now, let's consider the dangers when you eat too much sugar . . .

DIABETES. TOO MUCH SUGAR LEADS TO INSULIN SHOTS

I have real sympathy for any person who faces needle injections, day after day. Diabetics, taking insulin, are forced to endure this treatment—or risk terrible consequences.

In the United States, today, diabetes is the third largest cause of death. The other two killers are cardiovascular disease and cancer.

Grim statistics also prove that vast numbers of Americans are now losing their fight against diabetes. Because of this illness, they require surgery. It's a shocking fact that each year there are 60,000 leg amputations performed.

This gruesome toll of limbs is just one tragic result of diabetes. Across America, this same disease is the leading cause of blindness.

We know why people develop diabetes. The sugar chemistry of their body has been upset. The amount of glucose in their blood will vary—*depending on what the patient eats,* their blood sugar level will rise abnormally.

Diabetes is one ailment which is *diet-related* . . . and most medical doctors immediately warn their patients to change their eating habits. "Reduce your intake of sugars, that's imperative!"

I have always limited the amount of sugar that is allowed in my dietary program. All the menus and recipes which I recommend for arthritics are low in sugar content. Therefore, my nutritional ideas can also be very beneficial for anyone who has diabetes.

Repeatedly, throughout this book, I have warned against eating too many sweets. Instead of sugar, I have suggested that you should use natural substitutes in most of the recipes.

The foods I have listed—and the proposals I have made as to *when* you should drink beverages—

were carefully designed so that you would place the least possible strain on your pancreas. That's the goal, for arthritics *and* diabetics. Protect your pancreas!

The medical profession agrees that diabetes is a malfunctioning of the pancreas. The organ is not able to cope with the amount of sugar which the digestive system is delivering to the pancreas. Therefore, the blood, in a diabetic, soon develops too high a level of glucose.

You will notice that my "Special Health Drink" (on page 126) includes Brewer's yeast. This product has often been called "the poor man's insulin"—it is so healthful for diabetics.

Specifically, Brewer's yeast contains a generous supply of B-complex vitamins. They can help correct the overabundance of sugar in a diabetic's bloodstream.

Many arthritics—as they grow older and reach their senior years—must also fight off the scourge of diabetes. I often hear from people who have both maladies, simultaneously.

By complete coincidence, while I was writing this chapter, my mailman delivered a packet of letters. My publisher, in Connecticut, forwards any mail which is addressed to me . . . and look what came in this week . . .

This is the actual correspondence . . .

It is from a nice lady, who was the victim of two illnesses. She wrote:

Dear Sir:

I am sending this letter to you (the Publisher).

I want Dale Alexander to know what his program on nutrition for arthritis and diabetes has done for me.

I suffered severely for a year with arthritis of the spine, in my neck and up the back of my head. It was so severe I could not function well enough to accomplish anything.

By an act of God, I was presented with a book called 'Good Health and Common Sense' written by Dale Alexander. I followed the chapter on arthritis, taking cod liver oil, brewer's yeast, etc.

Within a few weeks I was much better, and, now after five months I am free of any arthritis. It works. All the drugs I took prescribed by doctors did no good.

Also, I've been a diabetic for 30 years, and I've had to use insulin. The brewer's yeast has definitely lowered my blood sugar. I've cut my insulin 10 units.

Mr. Alexander is a king in my book. I thank you, Dale Alexander.

> Sixty-one years old and feeling great . . .
> Signed
> **M.L.**
> **Viola, Illinois**

I truly appreciate those warm words of praise. They reinforce my theories about nutrition. I receive countless letters, unsolicited testimonials.

But, I am also a realist. No matter how many letters are sent to me, the medical profession will still argue that my dietary program is not valid. Doctors will say that my research work has not had any *clinical tests*. Gentlemen, just read the next page . . .

CHAPTER XIX

Believability. Are My Theories Tested Or Contested?

The title of this chapter asks a blunt question. And I intend to answer it. Publicly, and in print.

I know, full well, that my dietary program has been soundly criticized. Charges have been made that my nutritional procedure has not been adequately tested. According to *some* members of the medical profession, my dietary plan is an unproven theory.

On more than a few occasions, my credibility has been challenged. In the past, I have taken this verbal abuse, very quietly. But, now, in this chapter, I shall reply!

When my first book gained wide acceptance by the public, a storm of controversy developed. It was led by some rheumatologists in Massachusetts. They spoke out, from the Boston area. They spread their opinions, in an attempt to counteract mine.

The issue was whether or not there *was* any oil in the synovial fluid of human beings. The Boston doctors claimed such oil, in the joint cavities, did not even exist.

Unable to gather sufficient amounts of synovial fluid from humans, these arthritis "experts" were conducting their tests with synovial fluid taken from cows.

Based on bovine fluid, they were making flat statements concerning human arthritics.

On this matter——the type of testing——I'll let you decide about their credibility.

Perhaps they should not be harshly blamed. At that time, in the late 1950's, certain scientific equipment had not yet been invented to identify the oils.

I was convinced, of course, that these oils were a reality . . . and their effectiveness could be *increased* through proper diet. My first book also explained how and why cod liver oil was an essential weapon.

My critics prevailed, however. They frightened many doctors, caused them to reject the book.

Seeking support, I approached the American cod liver oil industry . . . urging them to test my theories in their laboratories. Supposedly, they knew their product and could scientifically prove its benefits for arthritics.

I was discouraged. My efforts to arrange a full-scale clinical evaluation had apparently failed.

But now comes the good news . . .

The facts I am about to reveal have never been told before. I saved this outstanding development—— so I could publish the *facts* in this book.

My dietary program *has* been tested, on human patients, with excellent results.

The clinical evaluation was conducted secretly——without my knowledge, and without any persuasion on my part.

It happened because thousands of arthritics, in

England, were reading my first book. Favorable articles began to appear in newspapers. Letters, from grateful arthritics, impressed some key scientists in London.

A study was commissioned, and the research work was done at the Charterhouse Rheumatism Clinic. A group of 103 patients agreed to participate, and the tests would continue for 20 weeks.

Dr. Harry Coke was the scientist in charge of all these experiments. With each patient, he began by aspirating fluid from their afflicted joints. With a needle, he withdrew synovial fluid from their knee joints.

The aspirated samples were sent to a laboratory in Hull, England. There, gas chromatography was used to analyze the lipids——*the oils!*

The chromatography equipment had been invented recently. (In fairness, I add that this scientific device was not available when the Boston doctors did their earlier research.)

All the patients, in London, had oil in their synovial fluid, from the very start.

As part of this clinical evaluation, the 103 patients were all given cod liver oil. One tablespoon per day, for 20 weeks.

Then, each patient was aspirated again. Gas liquid chromatography again measured each sample——drawn directly from the arthritic joints. The results were outstandingly good. In only 20 weeks, the oils had increased from an average of 0.12% to 2.58%. In effect, the patients had more than twenty-fold their supply of beneficial oils!

Believability. Are My Theories Tested Or Contested?

I am humbly indebted to Dr. Coke and his staff, for their diligent work. The evidence is now on the record. I rest my case.

That medical evaluation, at the Charterhouse Rheumatism Clinic, was later reviewed by other doctors and arthritis authorities.

One such expert is Dr. Verna Wright, renowned as a Professor of Rheumatology at the University of Leeds. Dr. Wright was asked to comment on what Dr. Coke had proved by these tests.

Here is just one statement made by Dr. Wright: *"The most exciting concept is that cod liver oil may be a precursor to prostaglandins."*

What a happy prospect that is! Other researchers, around the globe, should respond to that cue. The medical world is currently investigating fatty acids (prostaglandins) . . . and cod liver oil should be included in their future tests.

With my views substantiated, I shall continue my research work, more actively than ever.

The accomplishments at Charterhouse Clinic have sustained me, and I am most thankful for the confidence that they showed in my nutritional theory.

I have struggled, *for 30 years,* trying to secure some kind of support from rheumatologists here in America. My countrymen, I'm sorry to say, are still skeptical. I refer to those doctors in "organized" medicine . . . those who keep insisting that my dietary program is a myth, unable to help arthritics.

Until quite recently, they claimed that fish oil as a therapeutic substance was a fish story.

DIGESTIVE SYSTEM

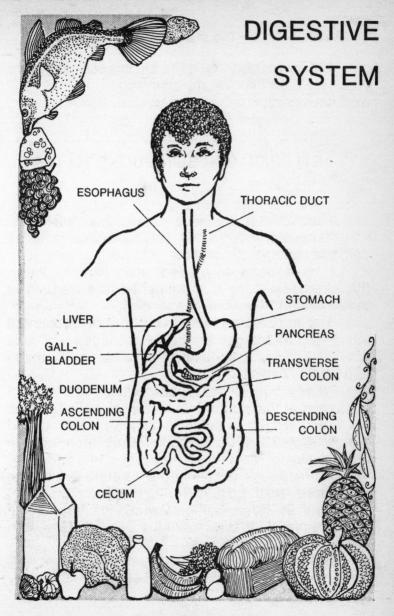

ESOPHAGUS

THORACIC DUCT

STOMACH

LIVER

PANCREAS

GALL-
BLADDER

TRANSVERSE
COLON

DUODENUM

ASCENDING
COLON

DESCENDING
COLON

CECUM

But, now, this year, there are encouraging signs that negative attitudes are changing. Very important experiments have begun—in Boston, U.S.A.!

AT LAST! RESEARCH BEING DONE TO TEST FISH OILS

Finally, after all these years, rheumatologists and respected doctors are starting to acknowledge that oil-bearing diets *might* affect arthritis.

I have been heartened and inspired anew, thanks to something that happened at a meeting of the American Rheumatism Association.

The foremost arthritis experts from throughout the United States gathered in Minneapolis—in June of 1984—to discuss the latest advances being made to treat this disease.

Nearly 500 medical papers and reports were presented at that conference. New scientific projects were revealed. One analytical study they announced is truly significant. Doctors, doing research work in Massachusetts, described their successful tests.

I immediately telephoned the Veterans Hospital in Bedford (near Boston) to seek full information. I spoke with Dr. Edgar Cathcart, who is in charge of the experiments. He is Director of the Geriatric Research Educational Clinical Center.

Dr. Cathcart and his colleagues, after months of work, accomplished a successful series of laboratory experiments. They set out to determine the value of fish oil versus corn oil—in regard to inflammatory diseases such as collagen induced arthritis.

(The expert staff included biochemists, a veterinarian, researchers, lab technicians—a highly trained team.) They used as many as 160 mice during these dietary experiments.

I asked Dr. Cathcart to describe the exact way in which these tests were conducted. "What did you do, as the first step?"

"We began by injecting a collagen material into the ears of the mice. We created an arthritis-like condition in the animals.

"The mice were then divided into two groups. One group was maintained on a diet which contained 7% corn oil. The other mice were fed the same diet, but instead of corn oil, we augmented their food with 7% of fish oil."

(The fish oil selected from these experiments was taken from a species known as Menhaden. This is a shad-like fish, caught off the Northeastern coast of New England. I just wish they had used codfish. I am a bit prejudiced toward cod, as you know.)

Dr. Cathcart continued his description of the experiments, as follows:

"After 23 days, we tested the blood of all the mice. Those mice who had been given fish oil experienced *better immunity protection.*"

Here was proof that dietary fat can modify the outcome of autoimmune diseases!

In the paragraphs above, I have purposely given

a simplified description of these experiments. I've tried to use non-technical language. Actually, these tests were very elaborate and scientific. From the mice, macrophages were harvested. Adherent cells were cultured for 24 hours ... the prostaglandins and the thromboxanes were measured by radioimmunoassay. So, this evidence is accurate, beyond question.

Yes, the medical profession is ready to agree that fish oils can favorably affect arthritis. The importance of marine oils is now being *confirmed.* The rheumatologists have authenticated these facts *in their own scientific laboratories.*

It's true that the experiments in Boston were performed with mice, not humans. But the day is soon coming when dietary tests will be extended to hospital patients. Human volunteers are certainly available—like those arthritics who took part when my diet was studied at the Charterhouse Clinic.

Throughout the United States, people are now eating more fish than ever before. This, too, is a very good omen for the health of our nation.

I have always recommended fish as a food. Now, several prominent writers have proclaimed the many advantages, urging you to add fatty fish and shellfish to your own diet.

Recently, *The New York Times* published a major article listing the benefits of eating more fish every week.

HUMAN BEINGS REQUIRE THE FATTY ACIDS FOUND IN FISH

Cardiologists are now suggesting that we should eat fatty fish and shellfish at least three times a week. This would have a protective effect on our hearts and blood vessels.

I agree. Occasional meals, featuring fish, can help lower your cholesterol level. Therefore, you will have less risk of blood clots. Minimize your chances of having a stroke.

The special report in *The New York Times*—in their column on Personal Health——was primarily written for readers who had cardiovascular problems.

May I remind you, however, that arthritics are closely involved. Most people who have osteoarthritis eventually die from heart-related ailments.

So, you should read these facts about eating certain types of fish . . .

Tuna is one of the fatty fishes which contain EPA and DHA, two very valuable fatty acids. I also recommend salmon, mackerel, trout, shad and sardines.

One 3½-ounce can of sardines can supply 40% of the daily protein needed by an adult. Salmon and mackerel are very rich in calcium, the bone-building nutrient which helps prevent osteoporosis. (For more about this disease, see Chapter XXI)

It is interesting to note that the Japanese have

rampant high blood pressure, but they have fewer heart attacks than most nationalities. Why? Perhaps it's because the Japanese subsist largely on fish—fatty fish that swim in the colder seas.

Shellfish are considered to be low in fat, but the fat that they do contain has a high proportion of beneficial omega-3 fatty acids.

Every year, the average American eats thirteen pounds of fish. But, by comparison, their annual consumption of meat totals 100 pounds per person.

If it is important to you to eat foods which are very low in cholesterol, then enjoy scallops, mussels, oysters and clams. They say "fish is brain food." So, get smart. Eat fish!

THE FUTURE . . . NEW METHOD TO TEST MY DIETARY PROGRAM

I have such confidence in nutrition—and in cod liver oil—that I am willing to cooperate with any group of scientists or doctors who wish to review my work.

Let's conduct tests, with human patients . . . *I am proposing that a formal clinical evaluation be made.*

New medical equipment has been invented in recent years. There is now modern technology that is even more accurate than the gas chromatography which charted the progress of the arthritic patients in London.

I urge scientists to use every device available, and every new technique, to prove whether I am right or wrong.

This is an open invitation to the medical world. Or call it a challenge, if you wish. Let's end the skepticism and dubious remarks.

Personally, I have already started to arrange a clinical evaluation—which could prove my theories conclusively. I am suggesting that actual *biopsies* be performed on patients who have serious cases of arthritis.

I am currently conferring with rheumatologists and surgeons, in California, trying to assemble a group of their arthritic patients who would take part in this *controlled study.*

Arthroplastic surgeons are certainly qualified to take biopsies—*while they are operating on patients* to replace hip joints or knee joints.

Yes, I urge that biopsies be done. In fact, in addition, let's examine patients with an arthroscope.

Joint linings can now be inspected, inside the human body, by inserting an arthroscopic device. It is a rigid fiberoptic rod-lens telescope. An incision is made (near the afflicted knee joint, for example) and the arthroscope goes in to look around.

This technique is a new one, totally reliable as a diagnostic procedure. The arthroscope apparatus was only an idea, a few years ago. Now, it has been manufactured as a modern scientific tool.

There are two Japanese doctors who deserve full credit for inventing the arthroscope. Dr. M. Watanabe and Dr. S. Takeda made medical history by giving the world such a valuable piece of equipment. It can be widely used, to benefit arthritics everywhere.

To gain added knowledge, a tiny camera can be attached to the arthroscope. Pictures of the intra-articular structure can be flashed on a TV screen. Now, we can have photographic documentation of how joints look. Let's compare the arthritic joints of patients who follow my diet, with those who don't.

Further, I propose that a series of tests be made by aspirating fluid from joint cavities. With a needle, fluid is drawn from the afflicted joint. My followers, who have been eating oil-bearing foods, will have synovial fluid that is clearer, healthier.

As final proof, the most conclusive test can be the taking of biopsies. A forceps can be attached to the arthroscope, which will enable the surgeon to snip tissue from the synovial membrane or from the cartilage. Give the tissue specimen to a pathologist, so he can study it under a microscope.

I am confident that biopsies will prove, beyond any doubt, that joint linings benefit from cod liver oil.

Those patients who have followed my diet will have better linings. There will be less infiltration of white blood cells. Less inflammation and less susceptibility to infection.

Perhaps then, the medical world will accept the logical truth. It *is* possible, through correct diet, to build up the viscosity of joint linings. Athritic joints can be self-lubricated . . . to alleviate pain.

Let there be no uncertainty, I am proposing that a *complete clinical evaluation* be made. A controlled study, using two groups of patients, comparing one against the other.

Take biopsies three separate times. Once at the start of the experiment. Then, 20 weeks later, the same patients would be tested again. And, to chart the lasting results, a third set of biopsies would monitor the patients a full year later.

As this chapter has shown, many scientists have made sincere efforts to authenticate my theories. I am most grateful to them ... and I pledge to you that testing *will continue.*

Any "new" approach to help conquer any disease is questioned, at first. And that's how it should be. I offer full cooperation to medical authorities. Test my dietary program on actual patients. I have abiding faith in the results ... past, present, and future.

CHAPTER XX

New Medical Discoveries . . . Some Encouraging News

While I was toiling in the field of nutrition, other men and women were achieving significant progress in scientific laboratories. Their accomplishments deserve worldwide attention.

This chapter will express my admiration for those unsung heroes . . . they are conducting experiments, night and day, yet their efforts are seldom known to the public.

You, as an arthritic, ought to be told about their research work. Your life and well-being will be vitally affected by these medical pioneers.

For example, do you realize the full impact of the recent discoveries made by immunologists?

Very few people understand "the immune system" which exists in the human body. It is hard to read any newspaper article which talks about "the biology of suppressor T-cells" or "the immunological value of antibodies."

Perhaps I can clarify some of this technical language. Because your future health may be changed dramatically by T-cell and B-cell research. The tests are being done, now . . . and the news is heartening for all arthritics.

254

New Medical Discoveries . . . Some Encouraging News

Just remember one fact: inside your body, you have approximately *one trillion* white blood cells. About 100,000,000,000,000,000 are antibody molecules.

The letter "T" stands for thymus—the thymus gland which manufactures T-cells. This gland is a small organ, located behind your breastbone.

The human body also has other lymphocytes which are called B-cells. "B" for bone marrow, where these cells are made.

When a virus or harmful bacteria invade your body, both the T-cells and B-cells react. They produce antibodies to "kill" the invader.

For instance, let's use the example of crippling rheumatoid arthritis. When a hip joint or knee joint is becoming inflamed (and then infected) your T-cells and B-cells try to counteract that distress. The cells "make" specific antibodies for that portion of your body. *If you have been eating properly,* your system can manufacture *enough* antibodies to save your health.

This is the viewpoint I am trying to impart to scientists everywhere. I respect them, for the research they are doing on T-cells and B-cells. But I wish they would place more emphasis on the patient's diet.

For more information on your immune system—and what discoveries are being made in laboratories—refer back to page 52 of this book. Reveiw the current progress which is now underway at the Research Institute of Scripps Clinic.

Twenty-six doctors and scientists at that clinic

are hard at work——seeking answers through immunology. On their staff, they have 190 research support personnel. The Division of Rheumatology Research is now directed by Dr. Eng Tan. This scholarly group is on the verge of making history for arthritics.

CHELATION THERAPY . . . PROVEN SUCCESS IN RECENT YEARS

At first, many Americans were hesitant to try chelation therapy. Now, the "newness" has worn off . . . and patients know that it is a safe procedure. If you suffer from certain illnesses, chelation could be an effective defense.

Numerous magazine articles have made the public very aware of chelation. In recent years, more than 3,000,000 treatments have been given. Patients have responded favorably, and many doctors now use this method to combat heart disease, diabetes and hardening of the arteries.

I believe that chelation can also be of benefit to arthritics. In these next few paragraphs, I'll tell you why.

Stated in simple terms, chelation is a modern technique in which a man-made amino acid is given intravenously. A fluid containing EDTA is infused into the patient. It helps to remove toxic metals from your body. The procedure causes you to excrete harmful elements, as you urinate.

EDTA is an amino acid which is similar to those

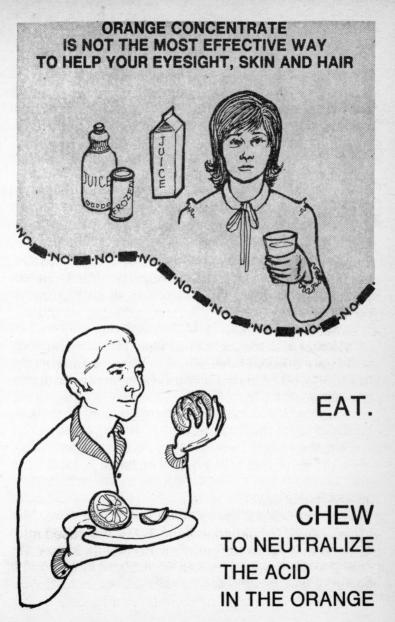

New Medical Discoveries . . . Some Encouraging News

forming protein foods. The initials stand for *e*thylene *d*iamine *t*etracetic *a*cid.

It has been proven, to my satisfacation, that chelation treatments can *de-sludge the blood*. This will allow nutrients from food to reach the joint tissues. Therefore, this result can be of real value in helping to relieve arthritis.

I am currently discussing the advantages of chelation with Dr. E.W. McDonagh of Kansas City.

Dr. McDonagh has administered chelation therapy for 21 years. He *knows* this field of medicine . . . he has treated more than 18,000 patients in Missouri. His chelation clinic is the largest in the United States, and he is President of the American Academy of Preventive Medicine.

On many points, Dr. McDonagh and I agree. Not long ago, I attended a lecture which he gave. As one of his key precepts, he stated: *"Balanced diet is the basic, down-home beginning for chelation therapy— to keep your body healthy."*

(I would also add that patients should *chew* their food more thoroughly. See illustration, on previous page.)

Dr. McDonagh also deplores the way food manufacturers process and contaminate wholesome products. He says:

"When raw wheat comes out of the field, that wheat contains at least 21 known nutrients. Like chromium, magnesium, and amino acids. But, then, food processors bleach it, grind it, roast it, and add a dozen chemicals and preservatives.

"After fooling with the wheat, we wind up with *only 13 nutrients.*

"So, I ask you, are we really making progress just because we are making foods more convenient?"

No, doctor, we are moving backward. Spoiling our chances for good health through nutrition.

Chelation may be a good answer for some of my readers. But, now, let me voice a few warnings about other medical techniques which worry me . . .

PLASMAPHERESIS . . . THEY'LL BLEED YOU, BY APPOINTMENT

Want to "flush out" your bloodstream, get rid of bad blood?

That's the theory behind plasmapheresis. Many arthritics have been sold on this idea—unaware of the risks and costs.

If you agree to plasmapheresis, you will find yourself being bled, in more ways than one. You may need as many as 30 treatments, with combined costs that could total $25,000!

Personally, I would back away from this form of therapy. Even the definition scares me:

PLASMAPHERESIS—Removal of whole blood from the body. Removal of plasma from the withdrawn blood, with retransfusion of the formed elements into the donor.

Allowing a physician to drain out your "old"

blood—so he can replace it with a more "healthy" supply—is a very grave gamble. I did read one medical journal which reported that *thoracic duct drainage* had been successful in the treatment of 12 patients with severe rheumatoid arthritis. But the dangers outweigh the benefits.

Supposedly, the purpose of plasmapheresis is to change the composition of the white blood cells in your body—to make them more effective in improving your immunity system. Then your body might be better equipped to combat viruses and harmful bacteria.

However, do the practitioners who perform this dire procedure ever warn you about the side effects?

Muscle cramps, lightheadedness, and nausea are apt to strike any person who undergoes plasmapheresis.

In my opinion, this "new" technique is close to the ancient art of bloodletting. King Louis XIII of France (way back in the 1640's) was bled 47 times in one year. And he still was ill.

I also recall the true story of the 18th century physician. He was known as a bloodletter. His name was Dr. John Lettsom. This is the inscription on his tombstone:

> When patients sick to me apply,
> I purges, bleeds and sweats 'em:
> If after that they choose to die,
> What's that to me? I Lettsom.

We can smile at his sense of humor, but the modern procedure of plasmapheresis is not a matter to joke about. Arthritis authorities warn that this periodic filtering of blood is fraught with serious complications.

To close this topic, let me quote an eminent professor from the Tulane University School of Medicine. Dr. Chi Shun Feng is also active in the Hemotherapy Department at Charity Hospital in New Orleans.

Dr. Feng declares: "Contrary to general belief, plasmapheresis is not an entirely benign procedure. Reports of morbidity and mortality associated with it are not infrequent."

For some ailments, as much as three liters of blood are "exchanged" in each plasmapheresis. That's a blood-curdling prospect for any patient to face. With all these worries in advance, here is a real instance where the "cure" is worse than the disease.

INJECTIONS FOR ARTHRITIS . . . A HISTORY OF FAILURE

Arthritis has never been "cured" by any type of needle injections——no matter what serum that needle contained!

Long ago, in 1949, they tried sticking you with cortisone.

Then, when that didn't work miracles, in 1951 doctors filled the needle with hydrocortisone. That practice has subsided in recent years——because the injections also caused a rash of harmful side effects.

Still, many doctors are experimenting with new serums. Currently, physicians are using sodium benzyl salicylate and even benzyl salicylate. By injecting these analgesics directly into inflamed joints, they *hope* to relieve pain.

I believe that these latest antics are also doomed to failure. Salicylates, which are actually just a liquid form of aspirin, do nothing to keep your joints from degenerating. Your arthritis continues to develop, despite injectable pain relievers.

Trying to stop arthritis with a syringe—by pumping some highly-touted fluid into joint tissues— is a worldwide mistake. In Europe, doctors are doing intra-articular injections with osmic acid and radioisotopes. The results are equally disappointing.

If you have arthritis, most anywhere in your body, you may be subjected to needling. American physicians have tried injections of corticosteroids in the knee, shoulder, elbow, wrist, ankle, and in the small joints of the hands and feet.

My advice: skip this therapy, if you can.

The third and last medical procedure which I want to warn you about is so radical that it's almost bizarre. Yet, many arthritics have been told they should try this treatment . . .

INTESTINAL BYPASS OPERATIONS . . . TOO SEVERE!

Some people with arthritis are also overweight. They have a condition which is now called "morbid obesity" . . . and surgery is one purported way to end this affliction.

Can you imagine having an intestinal bypass, just to lose those extra pounds! In recent years, we have all heard about the heart "bypass" . . . this has now become a favorite option for cardiovascular patients. Even double and triple bypass operations are quite common these days.

But don't listen to anyone who proposes that you have an intestinal bypass. The surgeon would perform this technique on your ileum—the last part of your small intestine. All this, just to combat obesity?

A better way to control your weight is through proper diet. It would be far easier to follow the menus in this book . . . much more pleasant.

Let me add that a study was done, among actual patients, in 1982. I have read the report, entitled "Rheumatoid Arthritis Following The Reactive Arthritis Of Bypass Disease."

In this report, the doctors had to admit one devastating fact. Nine of the patients came down with rheumatoid arthritis *after* the operation!

THESE BETTER TASTING OILS ARE NOW AVAILABLE

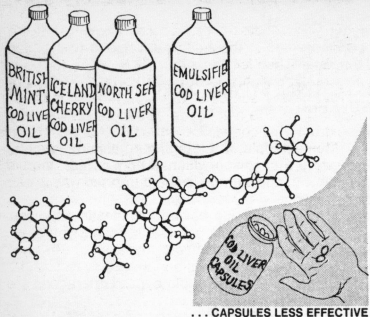

. . . CAPSULES LESS EFFECTIVE

A SAFE AND SANE REMEDY . . . THE OLD RELIABLE!

Why are we discussing new and extreme measures, like bypass surgery, when the best answer to arthritis is readily available in your own home?

Cod liver oil is the natural product which can

trigger your recovery. You already know it is not a new discovery . . . the medicinal value of this oil has been established for centuries.

Throughout this book, I have sung the praises of cod liver oil as a source of vitamins. Now, in the next chapter, I want to emphasize one more reason why this extract from codfish can improve your health.

My next topic, in Chapter XXI, is osteoporosis. For people who have weakened bones, cod liver oil can help you maintain *the correct balance of calcium and phosphorus in your body.*

CHAPTER XXI

When Bones Begin To Break . . . That's Osteoporosis!

Every time you visit a convalescent home, you can't help but notice the many people in wheelchairs. And your heart goes out to all those elderly inmates who are walking with crutches.

Brittle bones have become broken bones. It is estimated that *once you have passed the age of 60, then 90% of all fractures are due to osteoporosis.*

Many victims of hip fractures soon develop other complications—shock, hemorrhaging, etc.—which prove fatal. In fact, osteoporosis has now become the 12th leading cause of death in the United States.

Some scientists, at the Mayo Clinic, now believe that two types of osteoporosis exist. They categorize the illness by age group.

Among women, from 50 to 65 years of age, it is known as *post menopausal osteoporosis.*

Men and women, over the age of 75, suffer from *senile osteoporosis.*

In all cases, the affliction affects a person's skeletal structure . . . it is a deficiency of bone mass. Loss of calcium, in older people, leads to thinning of the bones and increased fragility.

Young people, when they are barely 20 years

old, make dietary mistakes. This disease really starts to develop at that early age. Prevention is possible, if you read these next few pages . . .

While writing this book, I had an opportunity to watch a certain television program on the subject of osteoporosis.

The telecast featured two doctors, both of whom are highly educated in regard to this illness. I have known Dr. Arnold Pike for more than 20 years. He is the TV host and commentator who is seen every week on stations coast to coast. Dr. Pike holds a half-hour discussion——on topics of health——with guests from every field of medicine. It is called "CAMPUS PRO-FILE."

Dr. Pike, himself, is Director of the Academy of Nutritional Sciences. His TV program is shown in Los Angeles (ABC-TV, Channel 7). (I have appeared on his telecast several times——to report my research findings on arthritis.)

Recently, one entire program conducted by Dr. Pike was devoted to a special interview with an expert on osteoporosis. This distinguished guest was Dr. Frank W. Varese. This renowned Italian physician received his M.D. at the University of Bologna.

Dr. Varese came to America in 1968, and he has been practicing internal medicine in this country ever since. He is now a member of the American Academy of Medical Preventics.

(Incidentally, here and now, I would like to praise the work of that Academy. They are a group of 500 physicians——doing excellent work. They study chronic degenerative diseases of the circulatory system. Their emphasis is on both prevention and treatment. Dr. Varese is particularly interested in osteoporosis.)

When Dr. Varese and Dr. Pike met, on the air, the telecast about osteoporosis was a very scholarly interview. They covered all aspects of this ailment, in concise language.

Here are some highlights . . . actual quotes, which Dr. Pike provided to me, as transcribed from the sound track of the television dialogue:

DR. VARESE: Osteoporosis is a very insidious and frequently crippling disease. It is the most common metabolic disease of the bones.

In lay language, we call it "thinning of bones."

Many experts in the medical field like to speak of osteoporosis as "the silent disease." Silent, because in many instances a patient has no symptoms whatsoever. The first symptom may be a fracture, a hip fracture.

DR. PIKE: What's happening to the bones, in osteoporosis?

DR. VARESE: It's a wasting problem. Bones lose substance, lose mass. A patient can lose as much as 40% to 50% of the total bone mass.

Why? The usual and normal metabolism of bones is disturbed, due to multifactorial problems—having to do with nutrition, with hormones, life style. Therefore, these bones become weaker, thinner, and frequently collapse. We have a fracture of the vertebrae, fracture of the wrist bone, or fracture of the hip bone.

Dr. Pike: We see a loss of calcium to bones?

Dr. Varese: Yes, there is a loss of calcium. Therefore, bones are not able to give support to the body, and they fracture easily.

Dr. Pike: Why does this occur so commonly as we grow older?

Dr. Varese: As we get older, everything occurs more commonly. Osteoporosis actually begins at age 20, and we see the evidence of the disease in older people.

For instance, in women alone (of age 45 and older) every year *200,000* suffer fractures—and, of these, 45,000 die as a consequence.

It is a total disease, for instance, when you discuss cost. Medical expenses, for the fracture of a hip, *for the first seven days* can be as high as $14,000! That doesn't take into consideration the follow-up of convalescent homes, physical therapy, etc.

Dr. Pike: So, the consequence of poor diet—as we are ageing—can be of considerable expense to you in the matter of your bones.

Considerable expense? What an understatement! Medical costs are so incredibly high these days, it's a major worry for every arthritic. That TV program, on osteoporosis, did not include any costs estimates for other forms of arthritis.

Suppose, for example, you have rheumatoid pains—to the point where you can suffer no longer. You decide to have surgery. Arthroplasty, to replace a knee joint, costs a small fortune! (Want to know the total bill for such surgical work? See Chapter XXII)

To escape an avalanche of medical bills—caused by osteoporosis—you need to know two main facts.

1. *Calcium* is the most important factor. Do everything possible to maintain high levels of calcium in your body. Eat calcium-bearing foods.
2. *Estrogen* is a hormone which can help reduce the "softening" of bones. Your body can manufacture its own supply of this hormone. Here's how . . .

ESTROGEN . . . YOURS FOR FREE, THROUGH PROPER DIET

For many years, doctors have instructed their patients to purchase estrogen tablets—this has been the prescribed remedy for patients who were fighting off osteoporosis.

Women often experience a deficiency of estrogen, especially after menopause. Scientific studies have shown that this hormone can sometimes prevent spinal fractures and strengthen bones.

Synthetic estrogen has long been used to reduce "hot flashes" during menopause. Now, in regard to osteoporosis, this same hormone can be beneficial. But why *buy* it? Why gulp down expensive tablets? It is a proven fact that your body can easily make its own natural estrogen.

Internally, your system can create hormones—including estrogen—in abundant supply. You can self-generate more estrogen with the help of Vitamin D.

Your adrenal glands are instrumental in making hormones. It is possible to stimulate your adrenals. They can be "triggered" into greater action. To learn how, see page 274.

RICKETS . . . THIS AILMENT IS NOT LIMITED TO CHILDREN!

Since we are discussing the whole spectrum of illnesses which "soften" bones and disfigure human bodies, I should certainly comment on *rickets*.

It has touched your heart and mine. You feel compassion, whenever you see a bowlegged child. We are sorry for the youngster who must go through life with legs that are bent out of shape.

Through the years, this affliction has been so common, it is listed in Webster's dictionary.

"*Rickets*—a disease of the skeletal system. Resulting from absence of the normal effect of Vitamin D in depositing calcium salts in the bone."

Medical science established this fact—proved the importance of Vitamin D as an antidote for rickets——during experiments performed more than 60 years ago. Working among children, Dr. Ruth Guy was a pioneer in this field in the 1920's. She was a physician, using facilities at Yale University. (See page 24.)

Simultaneously, another group of scientists and pediatricians were making headway against rickets——by conducting tests at Johns Hopkins University. Their efforts, in the city of Baltimore, were designed to prove the relative effectiveness of *cod liver oil* as contrasted with butter fat *for protecting the body against insufficient calcium.*

The experts at Johns Hopkins reported their key results in "The American Journal of Hygiene." The title of their medical paper was "Studies on Experimental Rickets" in June of 1921 and reprinted for a second time in "Nutrition Reviews," May 1984. Point: these ideas——theirs, and mine——are not a new, untested theory.

The medical team, in Baltimore, did a series of animal experiments. They fed groups of rats on two separate diets. A mixture of butter fat was added to the food eaten by one set of rats. Another set was given food containing cod liver oil.

Those rats which were raised on a diet that contained butter fat *failed to grow normally.* They developed a severe rickets-like condition. Some of them became permanently stunted.

Meanwhile, other rats were given the same food——with cod liver oil added. They stayed healthy, fertile, reproducing offspring.

The scientists published their conclusions;

"Cod liver oil contains a regulating substance which exerts a profound influence on the behavior of the bone corpuscles and perhaps on other tissues of the body as well."

OSTEOMALACIA . . . NOW BEING CALLED "SENILE RICKETS" . . .

Softening of the bones is the primary symptom. This illness strikes older people, but, in some ways, it compares to having rickets in childhood.

If your doctor suspects that you have osteomalacia, he will usually complete his diagnosis by taking a bone biopsy. He may find that the organic matrix of bone has not undergone calcification.

Serum calcium may be reduced. Your serum phosphate (your supply of phosphorus) may be decreased. And, your hydroxycholecalciferol levels are reduced to below normal levels.

To recover your health, how can you build up your body's supply of *cholecalciferol?* Remember the Illustration in the front of this book? The drawing of Vitamin D_3 emphasizes that this Vitamin is found in cod liver oil. The "3" following the "D" is the scientific symbol for *cholecalciferol.*

So, again, to repair softening bones, I am perfectly correct in recommending that you add cod liver oil to your diet.

DOWAGER'S HUMP . . . SHOULDERS STOOPED, NECK BENT DOWN

You have probably seen some poor woman who seems to be leaning forward, crippled into a painful posture, forced to stare at the ground.

The cause, again, is lack of calcium. Weakened bones. The patient has had continued collapse and crush fractures of dorsal and lumbar vertebrae. The areas between vertebrae, in the spine, have shrunken. As a result, the person has actually lost height. The victim, physically, is three inches shorter than ever before. The damage can be that great.

Take measures, now, so that "dowager's hump" never wrecks your life. Select your foods and menus more carefully.

For all types of osteoporosis, I recommend a specific group of foods which are rich in calcium. Remember, you must eat properly—to obtain at least 800 milligrams of calcium each day.

The best sources of calcium are:

Green leafy vegetables, such as broccoli, kale, and turnip greens. Egg yolk and soybeans are helpful. Drink milk, and eat fish. When possible, you should also eat the roots or tubers of the green vegetables.

———————

Earlier in this chapter, we discussed the need for natural estrogen. To "trigger" your adrenal glands—to make more and better estrogen *within your body*—you must increase your intake of Vitamin D.

The three most productive food sources of this oil-soluble vitamin are: raw certified milk, raw eggs, and cod liver oil.

Don't worry, you can avoid the "taste" factor. Modern technology has created emulsified cod liver oil. It is pleasant to take, literally tasteless.

For victims of osteoporosis *only,* I now suggest that you consume your cod liver oil from a spoon. Do not mix it with milk or orange juice. You should take one tablespoon of emulsified cod liver oil each day— 30 minutes before breakfast. See illustration page 264.

If you already have osteoporosis, that means you have drained the calcium reserves from your bones. It can become a life-threatening problem that goes far beyond the minor relief you can gain by taking *synthetic* estrogen. I repeat, make your own *natural* estrogen . . . as described above.

By observing my dietary plan, which I have set forth throughout this book, you can achieve good health. Otherwise, what happens? Turn this page . . .

THE MODERN DAY ALTERNATIVE . . .

ARTHROPLASTY . . . SURGERY!

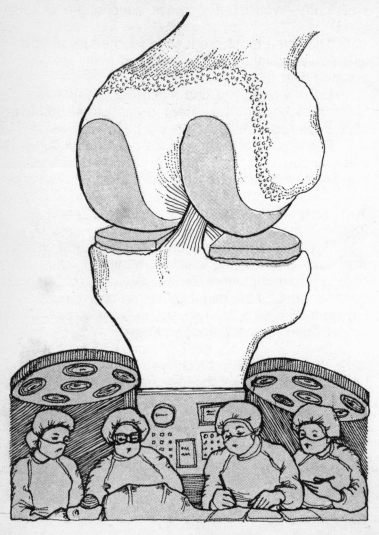

CHAPTER XXII

Surgery For Arthritis . . . The Price You Pay

If pain, inflammation and stiffness continue un-abated, you can't just ignore your arthritis. Don't sit around waiting for some miraculous remission. Either take some remedial steps, now . . . or you may have to telephone a surgeon and check into a hospital.

Surgery is a harrowing experience, physically and financially. Even so, many arthritics now subject themselves to major operations. For example, notice the illlustration (opposite page). It shows a knee joint. The grey area depicts a stainless steel plate, im-planted into the femur bone of the knee. The lower bone (the tibia) has a new plastic component made of polyethylene.

A successful operation of this type serves the arthritic patient in four ways. Surgery can:

1. Relieve pain in the joint.
2. Restore function.
3. Arrest destruction of the joint.
4. Correct deformities, and improve the appearance of deformed joints.

Yes, these are important advantages for a victim of arthritis. The success rate—for partial or total replacement of joints—has been high. Therefore, in this chapter, I shall give you the latest facts about this surgical procedure. You can then decide whether arthroplasty should be in your plans for the future.

I have known many individuals who were confined to wheelchairs. But now they are walking again—thanks to arthroplastic surgery.

Among all these case histories, I shall always remember one lady whom I met in Edinburgh, Scotland. *She had eight plastic fingers, two plastic hips, and two plastic knees.* She had been "reconstructed" so often, you might call her "The Bionic Woman."

Most important, this middle-aged arthritic was now living a happy, pain-free life. She attended one of my lectures, in Scotland, and I talked with her at length about arthroplasty.

Upon returning to the United States, I resumed my research into these surgical techniques. I am very favorably impressed by the post-operative recovery that arthritics report.

The future for orthopedic surgery is bright—as surgeons will be introducing artificial joints which are made of better materials. One expert who is predicting revolutionary developments in this field is Dr. James R. Klinenberg.

Dr. Klinenberg is a clinical professor of medicine at UCLA School of Medicine and is also chairman of the Dept. of Medicine at Cedar Sinai Medical Center.

The widespread acceptance of surgery for arthritics has impressed many doctors. Today, in America, there are more than 12,000 orthopedic surgeons . . . and many of them have become specialists in arthroplasty.

All these activities—the expansion of surgical aid for arthritics—can be traced back to discoveries made by one man. The principal inventor of mechanical joints was Dr. John Charnley. He conducted years of experiments, in England.

Surgeons, everywhere, credit Dr. Charnley as being the originator of modern total hip arthroplasty. He developed this medical procedure, emphasizing the low friction principle—utilizing metal against plastic to create an artificial joint.

The major part of his work took place during the 1970's. His contribution to medical science was so great, the Queen of England made him a Commander of the British Empire. He became Sir John Charnley, respected by rheumatologists around the world.

To write this chapter—in order to give you correct facts—I set out to find an outstanding surgeon who could answer my questions. In America, a recognized authority on arthroplasty is Dr. Leonard Marmor. In medical circles, his book is a classic. It is entitled: "Arthritis Surgery"—required reading for many young doctors.

Dr. Marmor, personally, has performed more than 900 hip replacements and 500 knee replacements. Today, he is attending surgeon at St. John's Hospital in Santa Monica.

I met with Dr. Marmor, and we discussed the latest arthroplasty techniques. We talked about synovial fluid, cartilage, the risks of infection, and a wide range of topics. I sincerely appreciate the way Dr. Marmor shared his wisdom.

How popular has arthroplastic surgery become? Or, rather, how *necessary* are these operations? To many arthritics, tortured by constant pain, surgery is the only solution they can find.

Today, far too many people must seek this form of help. Arthroplasty now ranks among the top 20 surgical procedures performed in the United States. Because of the frequency of these operations, that's a sad record to hold.

I was dismayed to hear that so many victims of arthritis choose surgery. To verify the facts, I contacted the Commission on Professional and Hospital Activity. This organization, located in Ann Arbor, Michigan, tabulates comprehensive reports from 1,600 hospitals across America.

If you want to know annual figures about any surgical procedure, this Commission keeps track of all operations being performed. Mr. Thomas Schill is in charge of the Commission's data base. I asked him to check the gross totals on arthroplastic surgery.

The answer: *More than 140,000 hip replacements every year!*

Equally grim——in terms of human suffering——is the fact that more people than ever before are checking into hospitals because they have serious knee damage. Each year, surgeons across America now perform *total knee replacements on 150,000 patients!*

These statistics concerning knees and hips are somber enough. But the bad news roster continues . . . and we must add all the operations on arthritic elbows, plus arthroplasty to repair crippled fingers.

FINGER JOINTS . . . MUST THEY BE FUSED, BY ARTHRODESIS?

I am glad to report that "freezing" fingers—so that arthritic bones are fused—is no longer done by many surgeons. That technique was fairly common until recently. But arthrodesis has lost favor, and more patients now ask to have their finger joints replaced. An arthroplastic specialist will operate on the patient—by implanting rubber-like inserts into the afflicted fingers.

We all know friends and relatives who have very painful fingers, inflamed by rheumatoid arthritis. Should they seek arthroplasty, the surgical solution? Many people decide to try this route.

To learn how much arthroplasty is being done on hands and fingers, I consulted the authorities who conduct the National Hospital Discharge Survey. (They are headquartered in Hyattsville, Maryland. This is a governmental agency, functioning within the United States Department of Health and Human Services.)

According to their survey, in a given year, more than 17,000 Americans are hospitalized in order to have arthroplasty on their hands and fingers!

That number of operations, while surprisingly high, also means that 17,000 arthritics have had the *courage* to face surgery. Medical science gave them a chance to lead better lives. Now, with implants in their fingers, their hands can function again.

We all should be grateful to the brilliant men and women who invent prosthetic devices like implants. More scientists should be doing work for arthritics. But they lack research funds! Read this next page . . .

Let's talk dollars and sense. How much should you pay to doctors and hospitals? What is a sensible price for arthroplastic surgery?

If *you* are debating whether or not to have an operation—to banish your arthritic pains—you must expect some major medical bills. On the opposite page, in a special Box, I have shown how our nation spends more than $44,000,000 on arthritis research. Now, let's consider the cost of arthroplasty to just one individual. How hard will it hit your personal pocketbook?

I decided to investigate . . . to do research, as though I were an actual patient, seeking arthroplasty. If I wanted to have my hip joint replaced, surgically, what happens financially?

First, I learned some encouraging news. These operations *are* approved by insurance companies. They *will* pay a substantial part of what the surgeon charges. The benefits paid will vary from city to city, depending on where you live.

FEDERAL FUNDS FOR ARTHRITIC RESEARCH ARE INADEQUATE!

36,000,000 Americans, Victims Of Arthritis, Are Being Shortchanged. The Bitter Truth . . .

When federal monies are distributed for medical research, ARTHRITIS is far down on the list. The total expenditures by the National Institute of Health are not being divided fairly. Here are some shocking examples:

Cancer research received $935,300,000 in 1982. That's an average of *$187.06 per patient.*

By comparison, arthritis research were allotted only $44,800,000. An average of *$1.24 per patient.*

What's more incredible is the fact that cancer affects only 5,000,000 Americans, while arthritis has more than 36,000,000 victims!

To find a cure for arthritis, a drive has now been launched to establish a separate Arthritis Institute within the government's National Institutes of Health. Let's all support that idea. It might help guarantee that research funds are distributed according to real priorities.

Even the public is confused. On television, viewers see a lot about Muscular Dystrophy. The annual total of money donated from public sources is *$74,700,000.* Some 200,000 people, with MD and related dystrophies, are affected.

Yet, public support for arthritis research (contributions) reached only *$24,500,000.* To assist 36,000,000 sufferers! We're even shortchanging ourselves!

I talked with the Health Insurance Association of America, in Washington, D.C. They reported that a person living in New York would receive an average of $4,379 toward the surgeon's fee.

Other facts they revealed, are these:

Average Benefits Paid For Surgical Fees

	FINGERS	HIPS	KNEES
Los Angeles	$1,154	$3,997	$1,906
Chicago	$ 933	$3,193	$2,563
New York City	$1,018	$4,379	$2,512

If you ever attended an actual operation, where orthopedic surgeons are implanting an artificial hip joint in a patient, you would understand why the hospital costs are so high.

The doctors and nurses must take special precautions, because this form of arthroplasty requires safeguards to protect the arthritic against any infections.

Pretend, for a moment, that you are a white-gowned observer, standing in the operating room at St. John's Hospital and Health Center in Santa Monica. Surgeons at this institution in California take most elaborate precautions to keep bacteria from infecting the patient.

The entire surgical team wears "space suits"— they look like astronauts preparing to walk on the moon. The hip surgery is performed in Laminar Air Flow rooms. Attached to the doctors and nurses are flexible hoses—which carry the air they breathe in and out of the operating room.

Sterile air is filtered and recirculated, and extreme measures are taken to maintain a "clean" atmosphere during arthroplasty.

These modern tactics—to defend you against infectious bacteria—cost money. The hospital bills will be sizeable. Then, you will need many months of aftermath therapy.

I know of cases where the aggregate bills for a hip replacement reached $15,000. Be sure to ask for an advance estimate. One tip: the fee paid to your surgeon should equal about 20% of the combined costs.

NOW HEAR THIS . . . LECTURE GIVEN BY A FAMOUS SCIENTIST

It was an historic speech, a landmark lecture on the topic of arthroplasty.

The talk was delivered in England, by Professor J. H. Kellgren, director of the Rheumatism Research Center at Manchester University.

He began by defining osteoarthritis in anatomical terms as "a softening, fibrillation, and eventual disintegration of articular cartilage, resulting in joint-narrowing."

Professor Kellgren then stated that "the essence of a good arthroplasty was that the resulting joint have a low coefficient of friction."

He commented about the use of intra-articular

injections as lubricants in "creaky" joints. The professor pointed out that "even if desirable, it was impractical, since the injections would have to be repeated with great frequency. *In any event, the joint fluid in osteoarthritis was generally of a good quality—that is, of high viscosity and consisting of highly polymerized hyaluronic acid.*"

As reported in the British Medical Journal, Professor Kellgren did not feel that muscle relaxants had any place in treatment, since, although the stiffness might appear to come from the muscles, *most of the symptoms arose from the joints and periarticular tissues, which could not be affected by such drugs.*

(I have underlined some of the quotes from that lecture by Professor Kellgren. Here, we find still another expert whose views are very close to mine. His facts match statements I have made for years.)

Now that you know the history of arthroplasty, you may have less fear of being hospitalized. Nobody likes to take that lonely ride on a gurney, into the operating room. But, sometimes, surgery is justified . . . and arthritics can gain dramatic improvement.

The surgical techniques which began in England (Sir John Charnley) have been refined and perfected . . . they are now widely accepted.

Patients now ask for arthroplasty, which is much preferred over arthrodesis. You should note and remember the difference. *Arthrodesis* is surgical fusion of a joint. Instead of binding an arthritic joint into a solid state, *arthroplasty* can restore *movement* and near normal function.

Your chances to gain relief will soon increase. Results have been good involving hips and knees. Now, research is underway whereby arthroplasty can be used for total replacement of ankle joints.

Total shoulder arthroplasty is also in the design stage. Early results in a few patients are considered encouraging.

In this chapter, perhaps I have sounded very enthusiastic about arthroplastic surgery. I do favor the technique——but I am not too happy about sending any arthritic to a hospital.

It saddens me when anyone neglects his or her body to a point where only a surgeon's scalpel can solve the problem. If you correct your eating habits, now, you can avoid arthroplasty. It's your choice. You can reconstruct your diet . . . or be reconstructed.

CHAPTER XXIII

Cholesterol . . . Some Conclusive Comments

Are you confused by the controversy which has been raging on the topic of cholesterol? I don't blame you for wondering. There has been a flood of newspaper articles—as many different doctors make conflicting statements in this "pro and con" debate.

In these last few pages of my book, perhaps the greatest service I can render to my readers is to write about cholesterol. Here's what I believe are the latest and most definitive facts . . .

The most reliable medical report on cholesterol—the one you can trust—is The Framingham Study. A total of 5,127 men and women between the ages of 30 and 60 (all residents of Framingham, Massachusetts) have been examined biennially for 34 years. They have had their cholesterol levels monitored since 1949!

For the results, worth reading, I called Doctor William P. Castelli, Medical Director, at the National Heart, Lung and Blood Institute in Framingham.

You can improve the ratio between polyunsaturated oils and saturated oils in your system only if you pay close attention as to how and when you drink water. In your battle to correct the levels of cholesterol in your body, please observe the water and beverage-drinking rules which I detailed on Pages 110 through 116.

Most adults, on the average, have a cholesterol level of between 200 mg.% to 250 mg.% per 100 cc's of blood serum. I believe that a better ratio would be to keep your level between 175 mg.% to 200 mg.%. Proper diet can accomplish this goal.

Within your body there are two kinds of cholesterol. One type is made up of high density lipoproteins, and you also have a supply of low density lipoproteins.

I maintain that you can and should increase your bodily supply of high density lipoproteins . . . and ingesting cod liver oil is one good way to do it.

If I were teaching in a college, a cornerstone of my course on Nutrition would concern the ill effects of water when it is consumed with meals. Everyone must be educated on how to protect the lipids (the oils) which exist in your body.

You must learn to change the function of these lipids. In the past, the emphasis has always been that lipids serve as <u>fuel</u>. In the future, let's learn how to eat and drink so that the lipids can bypass your liver and become <u>lubricants</u>. This is how to manufacture favorable prostaglandins.

As a foremost weapon in this dietary plan, I can again recommend cod liver oil. This type of oil can act as a <u>lesion-repairing</u> <u>substance</u> in coronary arteries.

In some areas, on the topic of cholesterol, I find myself in agreement with the noted nutritionist Carlton Fredericks. He is not in favor of the Pritikin diet, nor am I. That diet has claimed to build resistance to heart attacks by dramatically reducing cholesterol and saturated fat intakes.

Dr. Fredericks made some excellent points, not long ago. Writing in *"Let's Live"* Magazine, he said:

"Cholesterol is essential to life. Many vital processes in the body are dependent upon cholesterol, ranging from the sheaths (myelin) which insulate the nerves, to the manufacture of indispensable hormones, including sex hormones."

MY FINAL EXHIBIT . . . PROOF BEYOND QUESTION!

The mounting evidence which strengthens my case—more medical research that confirms my emphasis on proper diet—reached a peak in February of 1985.

The good news originated in Albany, New York, and I soon heard about it in a letter which was mailed to me from Newcastle, England.

Living in Newcastle upon Tyne is a prominent medical writer named Joseph T. McKiernan. I met him in 1979 and again in 1983, when he interviewed me for *"The Newcastle Evening Chronicle."*

One day, recently, he sent me a wonderful message. He enclosed a clipping from London—from *"The Sunday Times."* The headline announced that diet offers new hope to arthritis victims!

"Researchers have discovered that a diet of fish and lean meat, with fish-oil supplements, reduces stiffness and pain in the joints caused by rheumatoid arthritis.

"The discovery was made at Albany Medical College, New York State, after a rigorous trial in which neither doctors nor patients knew who was receiving active treatment and who was being given a dummy course.

"The results, reported in *The Lancet,* are the first scientific evidence that food plays an important part in the disease.

". . . The diet that helped the American patients is similar to that recommended for the prevention of heart disease.

". . . After three months on the Albany diet, patients had fewer tender joints and suffered less stiffness than others who had been on a standard American diet high in saturated fat. When they were taken off the polyunsaturated diet, the number of tender joints increased."

Let me express my humble thanks to the scientists at the Albany Medical College in New York State. They are recognizing some of the precepts that I have been preaching for 35 years.

This letter, from the medical journalist in Newcastle, I shall always treasure . . .

Dear Dale:

I nearly fell into the fire when I read the enclosed.

If ever a man was justified in what he said, against all medical opinion, it is you.

Let me have your comments for publication. In my
view, you have been completely vindicated.

Yours sincerely,
Joseph T. McKiernan

INCREASE YOUR I.Q. ON MS

It's time for all of us to learn more about MS.
MULTIPLE SCLEROSIS is a calamity when it strikes,
and this disease is spreading in nations throughout
the world.

MS, all too often, is appearing in patients who
have already contracted arthritis. I experienced a
shocking example of this trend when I was in Cardiff,
Wales, not long ago. I was being interviewed on a
Cardiff radio station. Listeners were telephoning
questions to me, on the air. That day I was besieged
with calls which all began with the same bad news:
"I have arthritis and multiple sclerosis! Why?
What causes this double trouble?"

The answers I gave during that radio broadcast
were crucially important. To help prevent MS, I should
repeat my views, now, in this book.

A person suffering from MS is also a victim of
dryness. Lack of lubrication, within the human body,
can lead to serious damage throughout your nervous
system.

Thanks to medical science it is now possible to
diagnose multiple sclerosis during the early stages of

the illness. (The method to detect MS is known as the E-UFA tests—an analysis involving Unsaturated Fatty Acids.) Glance again at the Illustration on Page 297. This disease affects the brain, the spinal cord, and nerve fibers in many areas of your body.

If you can hardly walk (and must drag either foot) that could be MS. You may have pain in your hand. That pins-and-needles sensation is one symptom of MS.

You might feel the effects of MS in your hand or foot, but actually these problems are due to damage which has occurred in your central nervous system.

Each nerve fiber is surrounded by a layer of "insulation" composed mainly of fatty material that is called MYELIN. Loss of myelin—through faulty diet?—destroys the ability of your nerves to conduct impulses from your brain.

This "drying out" process starts to happen in many areas of your body simultaneously, so physicians began to describe the illness as "multiple" sclerosis. Dryness sets in, then lesions develop. To repair these lesions, your body forms a crust or scar in your central nervous system. The term "sclerosis" means scarring . . . and no wonder your nerves can't function properly!

To protect the lubricating myelin which forms a sheath around your nerve fibers, start paying attention to the liquids you drink. Caustic beverages are your enemy. Defend yourself against MS, by correcting your drinking habits.

For example, in regard to this disease, I told

those radio listeners in Cardiff that their MS problems were aggravated because they drank too much tea. Those Welsh people imbibe too many cups of black and green tea . . . they demyelinate themselves with harmful tannic acid.

MS IN AMERICA . . . THE CITRUS SYNDROME

Senior citizens living in Florida often complain of painful ailments which could be identified as multiple sclerosis. Anyone who consumes copious quantities of citrus juices may someday suffer the agonies of MS.

Recently, I gave a series of four lectures in Miami Beach. In each audience there were people who had dual diseases—they were afflicted with arthritis and MS. To combat both ailments I urged them to avoid beverages which have a high content of acetic and citric acids.

In summary, I refer you to Chapter IX of this book. Study again what I wrote about acidity. Please review Pages 93 through 95, where I discussed the levels of acidity in certain fruit juices.

At one of my lectures, in Florida, someone in the audience asked specifically about apple juice. I replied that apple juice is a lipolytic liquid. It destroys fats and oils which your body needs as a safeguard against MS.

When you drink the juice of an apple, it goes

down too quickly . . . with no time to mix with your saliva. Therefore, your skin and your nerve tissues must neutralize the acid. Your saliva could have done the job, properly. The better method is to eat an apple. Chew it, thoroughly. Let your saliva be the neutralizer.

AUTHOR'S NOTE: To help more people escape the misery of multiple sclerosis, I shall continue studying this disease—and I'll report my opinions during future lectures. Much of my knowledge about this illness was gathered in personal meetings I have had with doctors and scientists. Among the experts I have consulted are two of the world's foremost authorities on MS. Next month, I shall travel to Great Britain, where I will meet with them again.

I am grateful for the insight which was given to me by Dr. Michael Crawford, a biochemist at the Nuffield Laboratories of Comparative Medicine in London. I am also indebted to Dr. E. J. Field, famed for his work in the Multiple Sclerosis Research Unit at the Royal Victoria Infirmary, Newcastle upon Tyne. Thank you, gentlemen!

CHOOSE THE RIGHT TRACK . . .

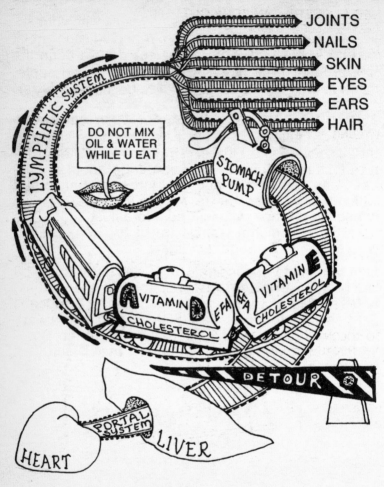

. . . THIS IS THE CORRECT ROUTE . . . SO YOUR BODY CAN MAINTAIN THE PROPER LEVELS OF **CHOLESTEROL.**

FOLLOW THE DIETARY SIGNALS SET FORTH IN THIS CHAPTER. HELP YOUR SYSTEN TO **ASSIMILATE** OILS . . . SO THEY CAN TRAVEL TO THEIR IDEAL DESTINATION.

CENTRAL NERVOUS SYSTEM

NERVE FIBERS CAN "DRY OUT"
THEY ARE SURROUNDED
BY A LAYER OF FATTY
MATERIAL KNOWN
AS MYELIN

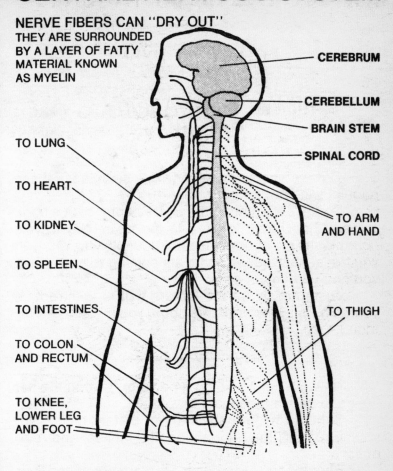

- CEREBRUM
- CEREBELLUM
- BRAIN STEM
- SPINAL CORD

TO LUNG

TO HEART

TO KIDNEY

TO SPLEEN

TO INTESTINES

TO COLON
AND RECTUM

TO KNEE,
LOWER LEG
AND FOOT

TO ARM
AND HAND

TO THIGH

LACK OF LUBRICATION . . . LACK OF MYELIN . . .
CAUSES DAMAGE.   AS IN ARTHRITIS
PROPER DIET CAN PROTECT YOU

CHAPTER XXIV

Until We Meet Again . . . A Prophecy

Our paths may cross, one day soon, so in these pages I will not say "Goodbye."

Today, I am writing the final Chapter of this book . . . and I now look forward to the future. My travels now begin, on another lecture tour. If you read, in your local newspaper, that I am coming to town, then you and I can meet personally.

Just stop by, at the lecture hall, and introduce yourself. As a reader of this book, you are already my friend.

Now, as I stare at my typewriter, I wonder what words to use in these last few pages.

Should I write a summary of dietary facts? No, you've read all the information, the menus, and recipes.

Should I say even one more word about cod liver oil. No. You've got the message.

Should I complain, one last time, about certain doctors and critics. Of course not.

In fact, suppose I end on a lighter note. I once

read a poem by Stephen Vincent Benét. Yes, he wrote some poetry about arthritis. These lines:

> You do not shoot the doctor,
> even when he looks perplexed,
> And you wonder rather dolefully,
> just what is coming next.
> From a weekly dose of gold salts,
> to a jacket made of tin—
> Just swallow down your aspirin,
> and take it on the chin.

I envy a poet who can write humorously about arthritis. To me, this illness is far too serious. Seldom can I smile.

America, as a nation, is suffering the results . . . arthritis is a costly blow to our economy. On the next page, you can read the devastating truth.

For you, however, arthritis is a personal and painful problem. If your joints ache, all you want to know is some method of relief.

I hope this book has offered you encouragement, knowledge, and some valid ideas you can act upon.

As for me, my work has only begun. There is more research to be performed . . . millions of people who must be convinced that nutrition is best. I sincerely believe that these pages hold the most practical answer to arthritis.

Perhaps, someday, colleges and universities around the world will teach dietary techniques to prevent disease. I'll make a prophecy . . . the day is coming when educational institutions will establish a Chair of Nutrition as part of their academic program.

Another prediction . . . by the turn of the century, my theories about "osmosis" and oil-bearing foods may become known as the Law of Assimilation. It may be accepted as medical fact.

Meanwhile, you now have all the facts necessary. You can make a beginning, or ignore them. But you know what? I trust your common sense.

ARTHRITIS . . . A SAVAGE FOE

Doing Tremendous Damage
to the American Economy

The financial impact of arthritis——the drain on our national treasury——is appalling!

How much does this disease cost Americans, every year? Would you believe $4,700,000,000? That's four *billion*, seven hundred *million* dollars!

Arthritics spend that amount just for medical care.

In addition, the price we pay then skyrockets to a horrendous figure. Just look at this bill:

$4.7 BILLION	spent by the public for medical care.
$4.8 BILLION	due to lost wages.
$ 1 BILLION	paid out for disability aid and insurance.
$1.3 BILLION	in lost homemaker services.
$ 1 BILLION	spent on quackery.
$ 1 BILLION	in lost income taxes.

The combined total——the economic injury to the United States, *every year*——is more than
14 BILLION DOLLARS!

What can we do to *stop* this raid on our funds?

We need an organized campaign to demand that more medical research be done . . . so our scientists can discover a *cure* for arthritis. Write to your Congressmen. Urge them to establish a separate Arthritis Institute, within NIH, *now*. (See page 283.)

For further copies of this book, and a complete list of other
Cedar titles, please write to the publisher:

William Heinemann Limited
10 Upper Grosvenor Street
London W1X 9PA